Prostate Cancer

Roger S Kirby MD FRCS
Consultant Urologist
St. George's Hospital
London, UK

Timothy J Christmas MD FRCS
Consultant Urologist
Charing Cross Hospital
London, UK

Michael K Brawer MD
Professor
Department of Urology
University of Washington
Chief, Section of Urology
VA Medical Center, Seattle, USA

Foreword by Thomas A Stamey

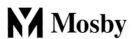 Mosby

London Baltimore Bogotá Boston Buenos Aires Caracas Carlsbad, CA Chicago Madrid Mexico City Milan Naples, FL New York Philadelphia St. Louis Sydney Tokyo Toronto Wiesbaden

Copyright © 1996 Times Mirror International Publishers Limited

Published in 1996 by Mosby, an imprint of Times Mirror International Publishers Limited

Printed in Italy by Vincenzo Bona s.r.l., Turin.

ISBN 0 7234 2050 5

For full details of all Times Mirror International Publishers Limited titles, please write to Times Mirror International Publishers Limited, Lynton House, 7–12 Tavistock Square, London WC1H 9LB, England.

A CIP catalogue record for this book is available from the British Library.

Library of Congress Cataloging-in-Publication Data applied for.

Project Manager: Linda Kull

Developmental Editor: Lucy Hamilton

Designer/Layout Artist: Ian Spick
James Evoy

Cover Design: Lara Last

Illustration: Dee McLean
Lorna Kinghorn

Production: Mike Heath

Index: Nina Boyd

Publisher: Geoff Greenwood

To Professor Geoffrey Chisholm and Dr William Cooner who dedicated their lives to the study of prostate cancer

PREFACE

The expression 'make it happen' seems set to become the catch-phrase of the remaining few years of this millenium, and it may certainly be aptly applied to those working in all aspects of prostate cancer. Virtually ignored for so long, this leading cause of cancer illness and death has seen an upsurge of interest over the past five years. The driving forces behind this are partly economic: it has been calculated that prostate cancer, together with benign prostatic hyperplasia (BPH), results in 4.4 million physician visits, 836,000 hospital admissions and 39,215 deaths annually at a health care cost of more than US$3 billion in the USA alone.

Moreover the ranks of those afflicted are swelling fast. Over this century in the West life expectancy has been increased by 25 years. Currently in the UK around 25% of the population is over the age of 60, and by 2031 this figure is projected to rise to 46%. The increasing numbers of men now reaching the so called Third Age (ie 50 to 75) hope and indeed expect to remain fit, healthy and vigorous. For them, over whom the disease hangs like the proverbial sword of Damocles, the argument that prostate cancer is a disease meriting low priority because of the relatively low number of life years lost carries little weight. Hence perhaps the increasing media fascination with the prostate over the past few years. This publicity has resulted in a rapid rise in the level of patient education relating to prostate cancer. This in turn has heightened the need for urologists and primary care physicians at every level to be conversant with the rapidly advancing knowledge in this disease area.

In this book we have tried to summarise state-of-the-art information about this very common cancer in as lucid and well illustrated a way as possible. Since in this modern world no-one, especially the busy practicing urologist, has time to wade through dense and turgid text, we have tried to make the book as concise and easy to read as possible, while still covering most of the important issues in some depth. We hope that this approach will be of value, not only to health care professionals, but also to the many hundreds of thousands of men around the world in their care who face the devastating consequences of this most prevalent form of cancer.

Roger Kirby   Tim Christmas   Michael Brawer

ACKNOWLEDGEMENTS

We would like to thank Dee McLean and Lorna Kinghorn for their tireless work with the illustrations. We are also endebted to Geoff Greenwood, Lucy Hamilton and Linda Kull from Mosby who have been so helpful in the production of this book. Finally we are grateful to Dr David Rickards FRCR for supplying many of the radiological images of prostatic cancers, and Richard Green for his help with the text.

FOREWORD

It is an honor and a pleasure to write a few words about Roger Kirby's, Tim Christmas's and Michael Brawer's new book on Prostate Cancer. So rapidly is our basic information on the natural history of prostate cancer expanding that it takes a lot of courage to write a book on this cancer. They have, however, done so in a most admirable way. For general urologists, and especially for internists and family practitioners (our new 'gatekeepers'), this book presents the dilemmas surrounding prostate cancer and how therapeutic options must take into consideration the unique features of this cancer: such as the fact that 40% of men have an invasive prostate cancer, but only 3% die from it; the extraordinarily long median doubling time for the early clinical stages of prostate cancer (4–5 years compared to 3–6 months for breast cancer); the availability of a unique serum marker (PSA) to monitor changes in cancer volume and grade, and the fact that the histologic grade of this cancer changes with increasing cancer volume, to name only a few important features.

The authors have utilized simple but elegant figures and superbly designed tables to emphasize the essential features of each chapter. This is so well done that the important message in most chapters can be simply obtained by reviewing the figures and tables.

All the chapters are well-organized; Chapters 2 and 7 are especially well done and worthy of careful study even by experts on prostate cancer. Each of the authors has brought their own personal expertise in prostate cancer and each has contributed to every chapter. The fact that three experts could agree on the contents of 14 chapters on prostate cancer is quiite remarkable.

The authors are to be congratulated for producing such a readable and useful text on prostate cancer. Their dedication of this book to two of the most gentle of gentlemen on both sides of the Atlantic – Geoff Chisholm of Edinburgh and Bill Cooner of Mobile – speaks volumes about the quality of all three authors.
Thomas A. Stamey, M.D.
Stanford, California, USA

CONTENTS

CHAPTER 1

THE

PROBLEM

Carcinoma of the prostate now constitutes a major and escalating international health problem. In many developed countries prostate cancer is the most commonly diagnosed malignancy in men, and seems poised to overtake lung cancer as *the* major cause of cancer mortality. It has been calculated that the current lifetime risk for a man in a Western society of developing microscopic prostate cancer is roughly 30%; the risk of developing clinical disease is about 10%, and the chances of dying from the disorder is around 3%. Risk factors for the disease include, quite possibly, Western-type lifestyle and diet, as well as the number of sexual partners and the age of first sexual intercourse; worldwide trends in end-of-twentieth-century living make exposure to these risk factors increasingly widespread. These, added to the well known demographic shifts towards an increasingly aged society (**1.1**), have led epidemiologists to predict a dramatic increase in both the incidence of and death rate from prostate cancer by the year 2020 unless effective improvements in prevention, early diagnosis and treatment are forthcoming (**1.2**)[1].

Unlike most other forms of cancer, however, not every prostate tumour constitutes a serious threat to life of the individual affected, and consequently does not necessarily warrant treatment. Many elderly men in fact die *with* rather than *of* prostate cancer, leading historically to some urologists adopting a stance of therapeutic nihilism for this malignancy. However, in the era of increasingly widespread prostate specific antigen (PSA) testing, such a position is becoming ever more difficult to maintain, at least in patients with a natural life expectancy of more than 10 years. In fact, the challenge now is to accurately distinguish those

Predicted demographic changes

% of Population
aged 65 +

Germany — — Japan   Year
Italy — USA
France — UK

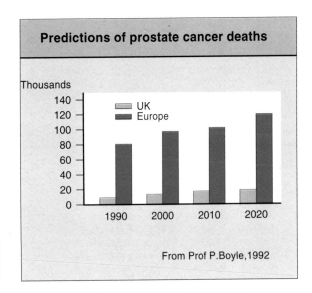

Predictions of prostate cancer deaths

Thousands

- UK
- Europe

From Prof P.Boyle,1992

1.1 Populations will age in all countries (OECD predictions).

1.2 Predictions for prostate cancer deaths in Europe up to the year 2020.

potentially dangerous lesions from the very small, slow-growing, well differentiated cancers that are unlikely to progress to present clinically within that individual's natural lifespan.

In this respect, current progress and future prospects are encouraging. Tumour grade and stage, in terms of volume of the primary cancer, have been shown to be important prognostic indicators. Ploidy as determined by flow cytometry can also provide important prognostic information. Molecular markers of tumour aggressiveness and metastatic potential, such as PCNA[2], Ki-67[3] and E-cadherin[4] expression, may hold the key to distinguishing those clinically significant and dangerous tumours that have been described as the 'tigers', from the 'pussy cats', which may best be managed simply by watchful waiting.

Currently, much debate centres around the lengths to which we should go to identify prostatic cancer early, i.e. at a stage when it is still curable. Few dispute that steps should be taken to diagnose prostate cancer in those with life expectancy exceeding 10 years who present to urologists with lower urinary tract symptoms. 'Case-finding' by digital rectal examination (DRE) and prostate specific antigen (PSA) determination in asymptomatic individuals, particularly those at risk because of family history, is also considered legitimate. Less consensus surrounds the issue of screening for prostate cancer – i.e. the formal invitation of all men to attend for a prostate check – since there is no evidence yet that screening effects a reduction in disease-specific mortality, and over-diagnosis is a possibility[5]. However, those cancers that are detected early by PSA measurement, the so-called T1c cancers, do appear to be of clinically significant volume and grade in more than 95% of cases[6], and are gland-confined in around three quarters of patients[7]. Long-term, randomized trials to evaluate screening and early diagnosis are currently underway.

Once prostate cancer has been diagnosed in a patient, histologically graded, and staged as accurately as possible, clinicians are duty bound to offer the best advice about treatment options, even though the risks and benefits of competing therapies have often not been formally compared in randomized trials. For the patient and his family, the decision concerning which treatment modality should be employed is often seen as a life or death scenario – perhaps one of the most important in their lives. Random assignment to a pre-judged treatment arm of a randomized clinical trial is obviously difficult in such situations, especially if one of the study arms contains a no-treatment option. In such circumstances, it is incumbent upon every urologist to be informed about all of the latest data related to risks and benefits of therapy, and to discuss these freely and frankly, not only with the patient, but also with his immediate family, so that truly informed decisions can be made about various competing treatment options available.

Numerous new therapies for prostate cancer are now emerging for which extravagant claims have been made, but their long-term efficacy in terms of cancer eradication and incidence of side-effects are still largely unknown. Interest of the general public in these new modalities, often fired by uncritical features in the popular press, is understandably intense. Androgen deprivation therapy continues to be the mainstay for metastatic disease and significant advances have come with newer LHRH analogues and antiandrogens. Alternative approaches utilizing, for example, retinoid derivatives, microtubule inhibitors and gene therapy also hold exciting promise[8]. These complex issues will be discussed and illustrated in greater depth in the following chapters; although we do not pretend to have all of the answers in this most perplexing of diseases, we have tried to set out the facts and controversies as clearly and concisely as possible.

REFERENCES

1 Carter HB, Coffey DS. The prostate; an increasing medical problem. *Prostate* 1990;**16**:39–48.

2 Harper ME, Glynne-Jones E, Goddard L, *et al.* Relationship of proliferating cell nuclear antigen (PCNA) in prostatic carcinomas to various clinical parameters. *Prostate* 1992;**20**:243–253.

3 Harper ME, Goddard L, Wilson DW, *et al.* Pathological and clinical associations of Ki-67 defined growth factors in human prostate carcinoma *Prostate* 1992;**21**:75–84.

4 Umbas R, Schalken JA, Adders TW, *et al.* Expression of cellular adhesion molecule E-cadherin is reduced or absent in high grade prostate cancer. *Canc Res* 1992;**52**:5104–5109.

5 Schroder FH. Prostate cancer: to screen or not to screen. *BMJ* 1993;**306**:407–408.

6 Epstein JI, Walsh PC, Carmichael M, *et al.* Pathologic and clinical findings to predict tumour extent in non-palpable (T1c) prostate cancer. *JAMA* 1994;**271(5)**:368–374.

7 Scaletsky R, Koch MO, Eckstein CW, *et al.* Tumour volume and stage in carcinomas of the prostate detected by elevations of prostate specific antigen. *J Urol* 1994;**152**:129–131.

8 Coffey DS. Prostate cancer: an overview of an increasing dilemma. *Cancer (Suppl.)* 1993;**71**:880–886.

CHAPTER 2

ANATOMICAL AND PATHOLOGICAL CONSIDERATIONS

INTRODUCTION

The term 'prostate' was originally derived from the Greek word 'prohistani', meaning 'to stand in front of', and has been attributed to Herophilus of Alexandria who used the term in 335 B.C. to describe the organ located 'in front of' the urinary bladder; detailed anatomical depictions did not appear until the Renaissance (**2.1**). However, while the existence of the prostate has been recognized for over 2300 years, accurate descriptions of the gland's internal structure, physiology and pathology have occurred only relatively recently.

Over the past decade there has been a flurry of interest in relation to the major prostatic diseases, i.e. benign prostatic hyperplasia (BPH) and carcinoma of the prostate. This is partly the result of the demographic changes (alluded to in Chapter 1) which have led to an increasing proportion of the male population attaining an age where they are especially susceptible to these disorders, and is also due in part to the introduction of a number of new diagnostic and treatment options in both of these disease areas.

Central to the understanding of prostatic pathology is a comprehension of the zonal anatomy. In addition, a knowledge of the capsule and the adjacent neurovascular bundles is paramount. These will be considered in relation to an illustrated review of the pathology of premalignancy and cancer of the prostate.

ZONAL ANATOMY

The anatomy of the prostate has been a subject surrounded by controversy for many years. The early descriptions of the embryology of the prostate by Lowsley suggested that the human prostate followed a lobar pattern of development similar to that of other mammals[1]. In humans, however, the dorsal, ventral and lateral lobes of the foetal prostate coalesce in the adult to form a rather homogeneous structure.

Subsequent studies by McNeal revealed that the lack of anatomically distinct lobes in the human gland was actually the result of an alternative form of architecture[2]. His studies used sagittal, parasagittal and coronal sections of the prostate instead of simply the conventional transverse plane. McNeal described three anatomical zones: the peripheral zone, the transition zone and the central zone (**2.2**). The peripheral zone in the normal gland comprises the majority (approximately 65%) of the prostatic volume. As its name implies, it extends around the posterolateral peripheral aspects of the gland from its apex to its base, and its histological appearance is characterized by small, simple, acinar spaces lined by tall columnar secretory epithelial cells. As is true of the entire gland, prostatic acini are embedded in smooth muscle stroma

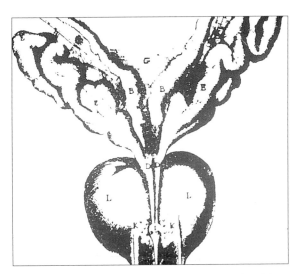

2.1 Early illustration of the prostate and seminal vesicles by Regnier de Graaf (circa 1660).

3

whose function may be to enhance the emptying of prostatic secretions into the urethra at the time of ejaculation, thereby allowing them to intermingle and liquefy with seminal fluid from the seminal vesicles.

The second largest component of the normal prostate is the central zone; this is a cone-shaped region that comprises approximately 25% of normal prostatic volume (**2.2**). The ducts of the central zone join the urethra at the verumontanum, and the direction in which these ducts run may render them relatively immune to intraprostatic urinary reflux, in contradistinction to those of the peripheral zone (**2.3**)[3].

The prostatic ducts branch towards the base of the prostate to join their acinar lobules, and recent studies have suggested different functions and longevities of epithelial cells in the ductal system when compared to those within the acini (see **4.3**).

The central zone surrounds the ejaculatory ducts and makes up the majority of the prostatic base. Histologically, the central zone is identified by the presence of relatively large acini with irregular contours, that are lined by low columnar cuboidal epithelium. The smooth-muscle stroma of the central zone appears rather more compact than that of the peripheral zone.

The smallest, but by no means least important, zone of the normal prostate has been termed the transition zone. This comprises only 5–10% of the prostate in young adults and is composed of two bilaterally symmetrical lobules found on the two sides of the prostatic urethra. The transition zone is separated from the two other zones by a narrow band of fibromuscular stroma which extends in an arc from the posterior urethra in the mid-prostate to the most anterior aspect of the gland. The ducts of the transition zone empty bilaterally into the urethra at the base of the verumontanum. Histologically, transition zone acini resemble those of the peripheral zone; the surrounding stroma is more compact, however, and is similar to that of the central zone.

The histological distinctions between the transition, central and peripheral zones of the prostate in man are usually difficult to perceive (either macroscopically or microscopically), because, in the absence of disease, their anatomical boundaries are relatively subtle. All of the mature, functioning, prostatic acinar and ductal epithelial cells elaborate both prostate specific antigen (PSA) and prostatic acid phosphatase (PAP). To date, few biochemical differences between the epithelial cells of the three zones have been demonstrated. The central zone *does* differ, however, in containing a relatively large proportion of epithelial cells containing a gastric proenzyme called pepsinogen 2[4,5]. Tissue-type plasminogen activator is also found exclusively in the central zone's epithelial cells. Epidermal growth factor (EGF) receptors also seem to be present in a greater concentration in the central and transition zones than in the peripheral zone (**2.4**), but the reverse seems to be the case with androgen receptors.

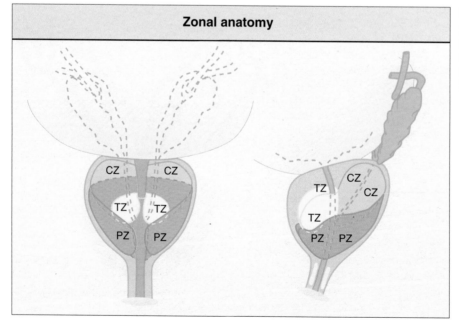

Zonal anatomy

2.2 Zonal anatomy of the prostate in AP and sagittal planes showing central zone (CZ), peripheral zone (PZ) and transition zone (TZ).

The clinical significance of zonal anatomy is important in terms of the development of both benign prostatic hyperplasia (BPH) and prostate cancer. Nodules of benign prostatic tissue usually originate within, and then expand, the transition zone; this expansion frequently distorts and compresses the adjacent peripheral zone. In contrast, although malignancy may affect any, or all three of the zones, the majority of cancers (more than 70%) are believed to originate in the glands of the peripheral zone. However, it is often difficult to pinpoint the precise origin of an individual prostatic tumour as this is obscured by the extent of its involvement as it invades across zonal boundaries.

It is still unclear whether there are distinct differences between those carcinomas that originate in the peripheral zone and those that form in the central or transition zones. Although it has been suggested that carcinomas in the transition zone demonstrate a lower malignant potential than those of the peripheral zone, recent studies have suggested that, grade for grade, tumours of the transition zone are little different from those that arise in the peripheral prostate[6]. However, the proximity of peripheral zone cancers to the neurovascular bundles may facilitate their spread along perineural and lymphatic channels (**2.5**), thereby enhancing their metastatic potential[7].

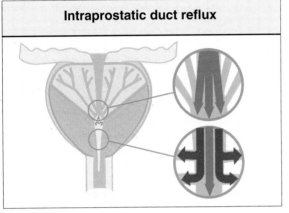

Intraprostatic duct reflux

2.3 The glandular anatomy of the prostate showing the tendency of peripheral zone ducts to permit urinary reflux.

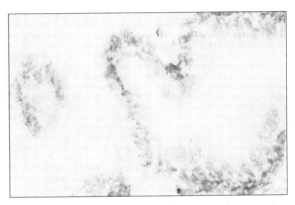

2.4 Epidermal growth factor (EGF) receptors in prostatic epithelial cells using immunoperoxidase stain and monoclonal antibody to EGF (×60).

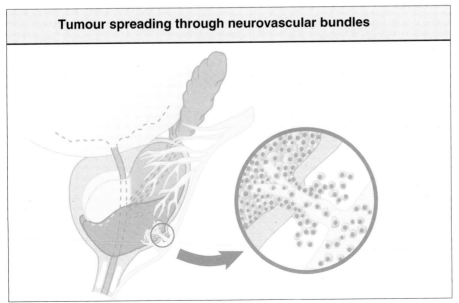

Tumour spreading through neurovascular bundles

2.5 Prostate tumour cells spreading by perineural invasion down the neurovascular bundle.

THE PROSTATIC CAPSULE

Long-standing confusion has surrounded not only the structure of the prostatic parenchyma, but also the very existence of a prostatic 'capsule'. Historically, the term 'capsule' has had two very different meanings. First, in glands that have been distorted by benign prostatic hyperplasia, the term 'surgical capsule' has been used to describe the residual peripheral zone that has undergone compression by the expanding transition zone; in this situation, the peripheral zone becomes atrophic and consists mainly of stromal elements. Second, and more pertinent to the study of prostatic cancer, is the question of whether or not the prostatic parenchyma is delimited by fibroconnective tissue similar to the capsule of the kidney.

The prostate develops by a form of branching morphogenesis in which the outpouchings of the urogenital sinus invade a bed of splanchnic mesoderm. The stroma organizes itself around the epithelial buds as they penetrate through the primitive mesenchymal cells. By the 16th week of gestation, the undifferentiated mesenchymal cells take on the differentiated phenotype of smooth muscle. It is this stromal–epithelium interaction which determines the ultimate borders of the prostate. When epithelial invasion ends, those mesenchymal cells within the range of their inductive factors become the outer border of the prostate proper. Mesenchymal cells beyond this boundary remain fibroblastic and establish the zone of loose connective tissue through which supportive blood vessels and nerves travel to the gland. The capsule of the prostate is therefore more akin to the adventitia of major arteries than it is to the distinct fibroconnective capsule that encapsulates the liver and the kidney[8]. As one would expect, the penetration of prostatic cancer cells through this flimsy capsule (**2.6**) appears to correlate with a risk of the subsequent development of metastatic disease; this will clearly affect prognosis and survival (**2.7**).

THE NEUROVASCULAR BUNDLES

The neurovascular bundles lying dorsolaterally and adjacent to the prostate carry nerve fibres and blood to the corpora cavernosa, and are critical to the development of normal erectile responses[9] (**2.8**). Their division in the original radical prostatectomy procedure

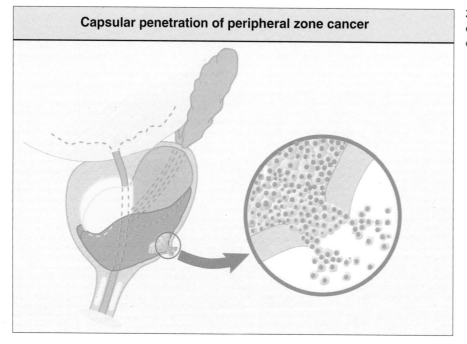

Capsular penetration of peripheral zone cancer

2.6 Extra-capsular extension of prostate cancer.

undoubtedly resulted in an incidence of post-operative impotence that approached 100%. The observation that these neurovascular bundles lie *outside* Denonvillier's fascia led to the development of the nerve-sparing radical retropubic prostatectomy described by Walsh[10], a procedure that leaves these bundles intact (see Chapter 9). Fortunately, this manoeuvre appears to enhance the prospects for post-operative potency, at least in younger men, even when only one of the two bundles can be spared[11].

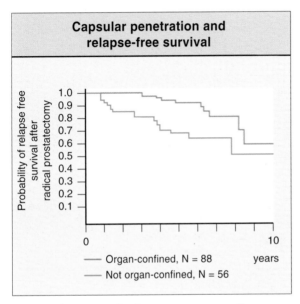

2.7 Capsular penetration by prostate cancer cells correlates with risk of tumour recurrence after radical prostatectomy. (Data supplied by Dr DF Paulson.)

THE SECONDARY EFFECTS OF PROSTATIC OBSTRUCTION

Prostatic enlargement from either benign or malignant disease generally results in a reduced compliance of the prostatic urethra and increasing outflow obstruction; secondary changes often occur in the bladder as a result. In anatomical terms, these consist of hypertrophy of the bladder wall, and the formation of trabeculae as well as diverticula. Upper-tract dilatation may occur, rather less frequently in benign than in malignant disease. The secondary changes in the detrusor muscle may be largely responsible for the most troublesome symptoms associated with prostatic obstruction: nocturia, frequency and urgency. The underlying cause of these symptoms remains controversial, but is probably, in part, related to the development of detrusor instability in the obstructed bladder. In animal models, obstruction to the bladder outlet results in detrusor muscle hypertrophy, collagen infiltration, and the development of involuntary detrusor contractions or 'instability'. A number of explanations for these unstable detrusor contractions have been suggested, the most plausible of which is an obstruction-related denervation, with the development of post-junctional supersensitivity to agonist transmitters. This is almost certainly only part of a complex overall picture, with other factors including altered adrenoceptor function, afferent nerve dysfunction, an imbalance of peptide neurotransmitters, as well as acquired myogenic deficit also playing an important role[12]. Whatever the explanations for the secondary effects of obstruction in the bladder are, it

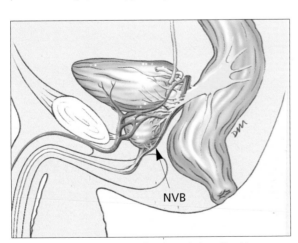

2.8 The neurovascular bundles (NVBs) described by Walsh, innervating and supplying blood to the corpora cavernosa. (**a**) Lateral view.

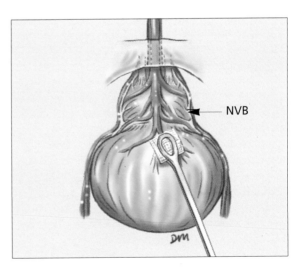

(**b**) AP view at surgery.

is clear that operative relief of either benign or malignant outflow obstruction can result in a reversal of the secondary changes in the bladder, provided that they are not too advanced and chronic over-distension of the detrusor muscle has not developed.

PROSTATE PATHOLOGY AND MARKERS OF PROGRESSION

The definitive diagnosis of any cancer demands cytological and/or histological confirmation of the established diagnostic criteria of malignancy. The prostate presents an exceedingly complex organ in this regard. A number of factors contribute to the difficult interpretation of pathological specimens from the prostate, including the large variations in normal histology, the changes associated with the frequent findings of inflammation infarction, and the effects of changing hormonal milieu; these are compounded by the myriad appearances that the most common malignancy, adenocarcinoma, may exhibit, not only between patients, but even within a given individual's neoplasm.

Despite these significant constraints, major progress has been made in the realm of diagnostic accuracy. Probably the most significant factor enabling this progress is the unheralded increase in the clinical material that pathologists are confronted with (owing to the increased incidence and interest in prostate cancer in general). Moreover, there has been a significant improvement in the technique of biopsy, which is the most common method of making the diagnosis of cancer; the use of spring-loaded biopsy devices (which afford excellent cores for histological interpretation) in conjunction with ultrasound guidance and a systematic sector approach, lessens sampling errors. The application of immunohistochemical techniques (which may help to establish a diagnosis of malignancy in equivocal cases, and may confirm or refute the prostate as the site of origin for tumours of unknown aetiology) has greatly assisted the pathologist in more accurate tissue interpretation.

As already mentioned, the greatest frontier in prostate cancer today is the ability to differentiate between those men whose prostate cancer is likely to lie quiescent (without significantly affecting his longevity or quality of life), and those who harbour more potentially aggressive neoplasms that necessitate radical treatment. A multitude of so-called 'markers of malignant potential' are currently being investigated for application in men with prostate cancer, in order to help stratify these two groups.

Methods of obtaining specimens for pathological interpretation of the prostate include core-needle biopsies, aspiration for cytology, transurethral resection, or simple open prostatectomy, as well as the sampling of lesions thought to represent metastatic deposits. In the US and now in the majority of other countries, the most common diagnostic specimen is the core-needle biopsy, which may be obtained by a variety of instruments. The spring-loaded biopsy devices, which are in widespread use, afford excellent tissue core, generally 12–15 mm in length and approximately 1 mm in diameter (2.9a–c). Owing to the low morbidity and minimal discomfort associated with obtaining biopsies with this instrument[13], multiple specimens are generally obtained (under sonographic guidance to improve the likelihood of sampling significant lesions), which, when cancer is encountered, effects a more representative assessment of the grade and extent of the neoplasm[14].

In a number of countries, but primarily in Scandinavia, aspiration cytology is still widely used. This technique, with its associated minimal morbidity and the opportunity it presents to sample a large volume of the gland, has a number of advocates (2.10). Excellent correlation with core-needle biopsy has been reported[15,16] in centres with a dedicated cytopathologist, but there exists considerable variability between institutions in the accuracy of cytologic diagnosis. This, coupled with difficulty in correlating aspiration-cytology grade with the more commonly used histological grading systems and the advances of the spring-loaded biopsy devices, has led to a reduced use of this method.

The normal prostate consists of an admixture of lumenal spaces, stroma comprised of smooth muscle and fibroblasts, with interposing collagen, blood vessels, as well as lymphatic and epithelial tissue. In the benign prostate, the epithelium consists of two cellular layers, one being of basal cells (flat cells with a horizontal orientation), and the other of luminal cells (which lie perpendicularly to the basal cells but have basally oriented nuclei) (2.11). The basal cells, whose function remains unknown, can be difficult to identify on standard histological preparations; however, one can readily identify this layer with high-molecular-weight cytokeratin staining, which identifies only the

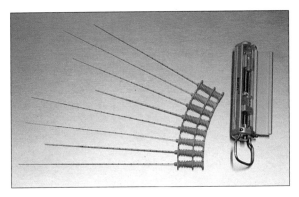

2.9(a) Transrectal ultrasound-guided prostate biopsy using an automatic biopsy device.

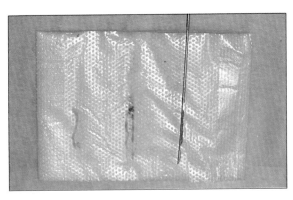

(b) Prostatic needle-biopsy specimens.

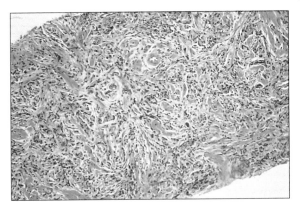

(c) Histology of a needle biopsy of a prostatic cancer.

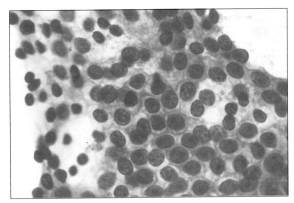

2.10 Fine-needle aspiration cytology: poorly differentiated adenocarcinoma. (Reproduced from Weiss MA, Mills SE *Atlas of Genitourinary Tract Disorders* Gower, 1988.)

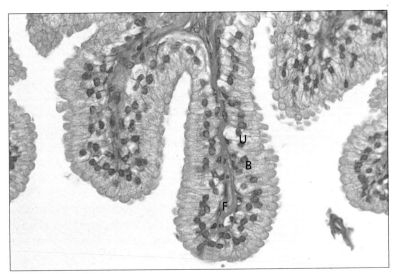

2.11 Benign prostatic epithelium as seen in BPH.
U = uniform columnar cell nuclei
B = basal cell nuclei
F = fibrovascular stalk.
(Reproduced from Weiss MA, Mills SE *Atlas of Genitourinary Tract Disorders* Gower, 1988.)

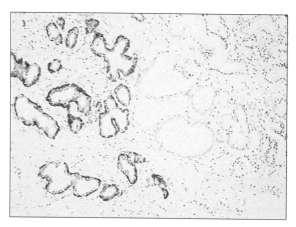

2.12 High-molecular-weight cytokeratin: normal (L) and prostate cancer (R).

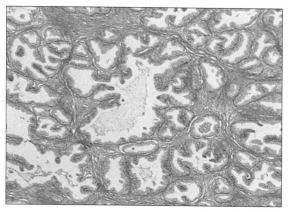

2.13 BPH – highly epithelial variant. (Reproduced from Weiss MA, Mills SE *Atlas of Genitourinary Tract Disorders* Gower, 1988.)

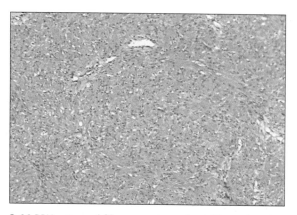

2.14 BPH – stromal fibromuscular variant. (Reproduced from Weiss MA, Mills SE *Atlas of Genitourinary Tract Disorders* Gower, 1988.)

basal cells[17]. This is an important feature, as carcinoma of the prostate is almost always devoid of the basal-cell layer, offering an excellent immunohistochemical confirmation of the presence of benign or malignant tissue (**2.12**).

Owing to the ubiquitous nature of benign prostatic hyperplasia, most men who undergo examination for prostate cancer will harbour histological BPH. A thorough discussion of this entity is beyond the scope of this chapter, but may be found elsewhere[18]. Histologically, BPH is an extremely variable entity, ranging from a highly epithelial variant (**2.13**) to a fibromuscular type that is largely devoid of epithelial components (**2.14**).

PREMALIGNANCY IN THE PROSTATE

The early detection and cure of cancer has often depended on the ability to recognize premalignant change. The definitive identification of the precursors of invasive carcinomata of the prostate has lagged many years behind equivalent organ sites, such as the uterine cervix. This is partly due to the technical difficulties in performing repeated biopsies on the same exact location of the prostate, e.g. when compared to repeating a PAP cervical smear or undertaking cervical colposcopy. Even with transrectal ultrasound-guided (TRUS-guided) biopsy, it is difficult to be sure that a given rebiopsy is taken from an identical microscopic field. For this reason, the interpretation of transformations within the prostate from dysplastic to frankly malignant states is handicapped by the lack of data concerning the progression of specific lesions over time.

Prostatic Intraepithelial Neoplasia

Progress in the area of identifying precursors was made in the mid 1980s, however, when McNeal and Bostwick[19] reported the existence of a lesion that they termed 'intraductal dysplasia'. This entity was proposed as a precursor of malignancy on the grounds of cytological atypia, exhibiting nuclear pleomorphism and nucleolar prominence similar to that seen in prostate cancer (**Table 2.1**). Following a consensus conference in 1989 the term 'prostatic intraepithelial neoplasia' (PIN) was adopted as the most appropriate nomenclature for this lesion (**Table 2.2**), bringing it into line with other premalignant lesions elsewhere in the body, such as cervical intraepithelial neoplasia (CIN).

In general, our understanding of PIN is based on its association with other areas of unequivocal malignancy. Transition-zone cancers are not usually associated with PIN but, in peripheral-zone tumours, PIN is frequently found adjacent to carcinomas[20,21]. Severe PIN is often more extensive in multifocal cancers[20]. Apart from the nuclear pleomorphism already mentioned, PIN lesions also share other characteristics of malignancy such as the loss of basal layer continuity[22], the production of acid mucin[23], altered lectin binding[24], evidence of differentiation as evidenced by decreased PSA immunostaining[25,26] and abnormalities of ploidy. **2.15** is an example of low-grade PIN.

The diagnosis of moderate-grade PIN (**2.16**) and high-

Table 2.1 Evidence that PIN is premalignant
Morphologic similarity to invasive cancer
Phenotypic similarity to cancer
Incidence is greater in organs harbouring invasive cancer
Severity is increased with cancer
Extent is greater with concomitant cancer
Spatial relationship to invasive cancer
Microinvasion present from the premalignant change
Progression to invasive cancer identified on serial biopsy*
* Not proven in PIN owing to 3-dimensional arborization of prostate epithelium

Table 2.2 Prostatic premalignant lesion synonyms
Atypical epithelial hyperplasia
Atypical glandular hyperplasia
Atypical hyperplasia
Cytologic atypia
Cellular atypia
Duct-acinar dysplasia
Glandular atypia
Intraductal dysplasia
Intraepithelial neoplasia
Intraglandular dysplasia
Large acinar atypical hyperplasia

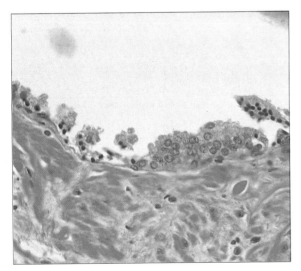

2.15 Low-grade prostatic intraepithelial neoplasia (PIN). (Reproduced from Weiss MA, Mills SE *Atlas of Genitourinary Tract Disorders* Gower, 1988.)

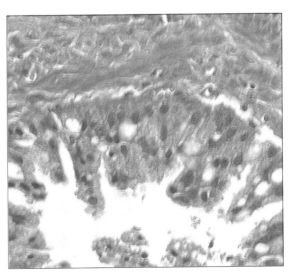

2.16 Moderate-grade PIN. (Reproduced from Weiss MA, Mills SE *Atlas of Genitourinary Tract Disorders* Gower, 1988.)

grade PIN (**2.17**) is established by increasing prolifera-tion and cytological changes. PIN is commonly associ-ated with disruption of the basal-cell layer, as identified by high-molecular-weight cytokeratin immunohisto-chemistry (**2.18**). This has led to development of a model for prostate carcinogenesis, which has become increas-ingly accepted (**2.19**).

Another lesion which has been suggested to repre-sent a premalignant change is atypical adenomatous hyperplasia (**2.20**). This entity, which is similar in appearance to low-grade carcinoma, may also be focally associated with disruption of the basal-cell layer. However, the evidence that this is indeed a pre-malignant change is considerably less definitive than that for PIN.

Pathology of Prostate Cancer

Microscopically, most carcinomas of the prostate are classical adenocarcinomata, being made up of epithe-lial cells with varying degrees of glandular architecture. As noted, there is a departure from the normal two lay-ers of cells (with absence of the basal-cell layer) which may be confirmed immunohistochemically. Addition-ally, there is an infiltrative growth pattern that often results in difficulty delineating the actual edge of the tumour. As mentioned, this makes the definitive site of origin difficult to identify in many cases (**2.21**).

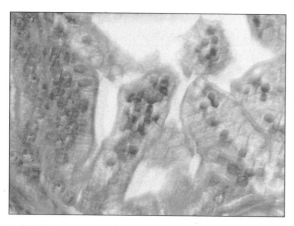

2.17 High-grade PIN. (Reproduced from Weiss MA, Mills SE *Atlas of Genitourinary Tract Disorders* Gower, 1988.)

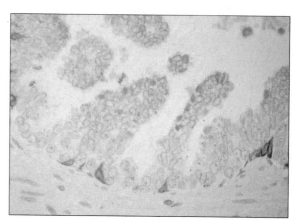

2.18 High-molecular-weight cytokeratin technique to demonstrate basal-cell disruption caused by PIN.

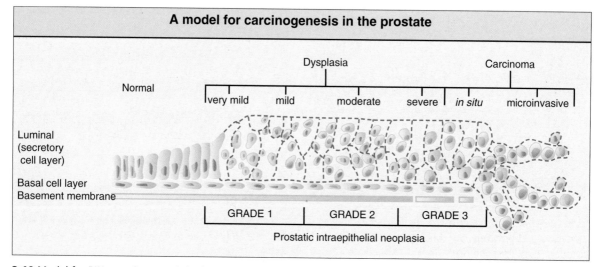

2.19 Model for PIN – carcinogenesis in the prostate. (Reproduced with permission from Bostwick and Brawer[22].)

One of the hallmarks of prostate cancer is the frequent finding of glands growing 'back-to-back' with no intervening stroma. Cytologically, prostate cancer is extremely variable but, in general, enlarged pleomorphic nuclei and prominence of nucleoli are found.

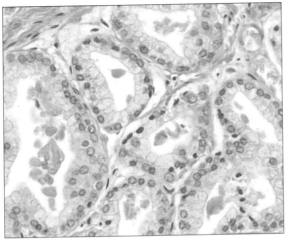

2.20 Atypical adenomatous hyperplasia. (Reproduced from Weiss MA, Mills SE *Atlas of Genitourinary Tract Disorders* Gower, 1988.)

Histological Grading

Just as in other organ systems, the grade of a malignancy or its degree of departure from normal has been established as an important prognostic marker in the prostate. A number of grading systems have been advocated, the most widely applied of which is that of Gleason[27]. The Gleason grading system uses low-power architectural findings to define the pattern of the tumour. A 5-step grading system is used, and the two most prominent grades are added together to afford the so-called 'Gleason score', which ranges from 2–10. **2.22** illustrates the architectural changes for each grade as described by Gleason. The Gleason system has been shown not only to offer significant prognostic information but also to be reproducible between pathologists[28,29].

Histological grading offers valuable prognostic information. Evidence of this comes from many

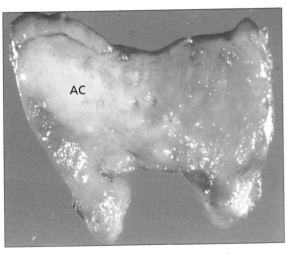

2.21 Gross pathological specimen showing prostate cancer. The site of origin is difficult to determine. AC = adenocarcinoma.
(Reproduced from Weiss MA, Mills SE *Atlas of Genitourinary Tract Disorders* Gower, 1988.)

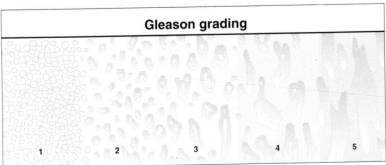

Gleason grading

| 1 | 2 | 3 | 4 | 5 |

2.22 Gleason grading system shown diagrammatically.

settings, including the most recent outcome of a meta-analysis of a watchful-waiting series by Chodak and associates[30]. They noted that grade 1 (Gleason score 2–4) had a 2.1% annualized rate of developing metastases; grade 2 (Gleason score 5–7) had a 5.4% rate and grade 3 (Gleason score 7–10) had a rate of 13.5%.

2.23 shows a Gleason grade 1 tumour comprised of small, uniform glands exhibiting minimal nuclear changes. This low-grade neoplasm, which frequently consists of nodules with well-defined borders, has been shown to be of low biological potential. The most common grade is Gleason grade 3 (**2.24**). This lesion exhibits the largest degree of variation in architecture, glandular size, shape and regularity; infiltrative borders are generally found. Gleason grades 4 and 5 (**2.25**, **2.26**) represent much more aggressive neoplasms with marked cytologic atypia, extensive infiltrative borders (most likely associated with capsular penetration), positive surgical margins, seminal-vesicle extension, and/or metastatic spread. Marked heterogeneity of the histological appearance of the high-grade carcinoma may be present and, at times, it may be difficult to establish the prostate as the site of origin, particularly in lesions extending beyond the prostate, either locally in the pelvis, or in metastatic deposits. The specificity of prostate specific antigen (PSA) as described in Chapter 6 on tumour markers, affords an excellent immunohistochemical test for the diagnosis of prostate cancer in such clinical scenarios (**2.27**).

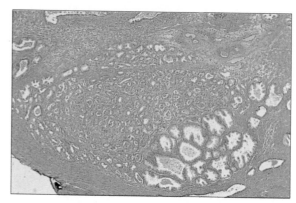

2.23 Gleason grade 1. (Reproduced from Weiss, Gower, 1988.)

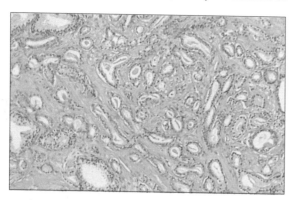

2.24 Gleason grade 3. (Reproduced from Weiss, Gower, 1988.)

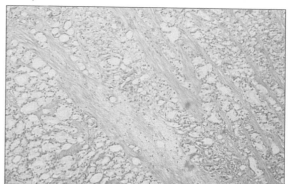

2.25 Gleason grade 4. (Reproduced from Weiss, Gower, 1988.)

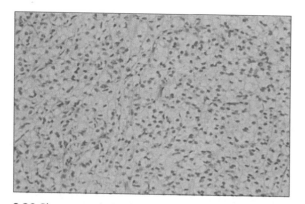

2.26 Gleason grade 5 infiltrating stroma. (Reproduced from Weiss, Gower, 1988.)

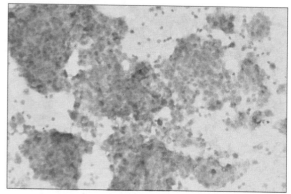

2.27 PSA immunohistochemistry. (Reproduced from Weiss, Gower, 1988.)

THE ENIGMA OF 'LATENT' PROSTATE CANCER

In 1954, Franks was the first to point out the extraordinarily high prevalence of microfoci of 'latent' prostate cancer in the post-mortem examination of men dying from other diseases[31]. Since then, numerous other investigators have confirmed this observation and noted that the incidence of these tiny cancers appears to increase with age; overall around 30% of men over 50 are apparently affected[32] and this figure does not seem to vary markedly between countries. Recently, a study of younger men dying of diseases other than prostate cancer has highlighted the surprisingly early age of onset of these pathological changes[33]. The low growth rate of these microscopic tumours (some prostate cancers have a cell-doubling time of more than 4 years) is probably the reason that they often carry little danger for the individual. A proportion, though, *will* enlarge (and also dedifferentiate), to a point where they become both clinically significant and identifiable by modern screening methods within the natural lifespan of the patient. The threshold of 'clinically significant' volume is currently regarded as 0.5 cm^3; by the time a volume of 3.5 cm^3 is reached, a high proportion of prostate cancers will have penetrated through the capsule[34].

The sobering statistics of the rising morbidity and mortality associated with prostate cancer must be balanced against the fact that the histological incidence of prostate cancer far exceeds the prevalence of clinically manifest disease. While perhaps 30% of men over age 50 harbour tiny foci of well-differentiated prostate cancer, it is estimated that only 10% of men will have a diagnosis of prostate cancer during their lifetime, and that only 3% will succumb to the disease[35]. Of the three methods for reducing cancer-related mortality – decreasing the incidence, improving therapy, and providing early detection – only the latter is currently at hand. However, an obvious problem exists with the widespread application of early detection or screening for this common malignancy: we may identify malignancies in some men who have little likelihood of a clinical manifestation of this disease, and who would actually be better off were their cancer to remain undetected. The overdetection of these malignancies, and the few methods of identifying those with a high propensity of causing patient morbidity or mortality, may lead to overtreatment. What are clearly needed in prostate cancer management today are reliable methods to stratify those malignancies that may well give rise to patient disease from those likely to lie quiescent. Considerable effort is currently directed towards the development of a number of potential markers of future biological behaviour (**Table 2.3**).

STAGE MIGRATION OF PROSTATE CANCER

The increasing application of early detection programmes has created what appears to be a 'stage migration'. That is, more men are identified with malignancies of lower stage and are thus perhaps more likely to be cured with conventional therapy. Recently, Ohori et al.[36] examined a series of men undergoing radical prostatectomy at Baylor School of Medicine. They classified the neoplasms into three categories (latent, clinically important, or curable), and compared these tumours to incidental cancers found in 90 cystoprostatectomy specimens. A total of 78% of the patients undergoing cystoprostatectomy had what were described as latent cancers (cancers smaller than 0.5 cm^3 with Gleason grade of 1, 2, or 3) which were pathologically confined. In 22% of patients, cancers were found that were deemed curable with significant malignant potential; that is to say, they had either a Gleason grade 1, 2, or 3 tumour with a volume greater than 0.5 cm^3 that was confined to the prostate, a grade

Table 2.3 Markers of malignant potential for prostate cancer
Histological grade
Clinical stage
Pathological stage
Tumour volume
Prostatic acid phosphatase
Prostate specific antigen
DNA ploidy
Nuclear morphometry
Neovascularity
Oncogenes
Tumour-suppressor genes
Invasion markers (e.g. cathepsin, collagenase)
Cell adhesion factors
Basement membrane (collagen)

Volume distribution of 100 prostate tumours

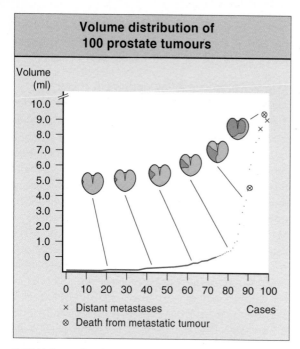

× Distant metastases
⊗ Death from metastatic tumour

2.28 Volume distribution of 100 prostate cancers in rank order. Only those with volume >1.5 cm^3 had metastasized. (Modified from McNeal *et al. Lancet* 1986[34].)

Seminal-vesicle involvement and survival

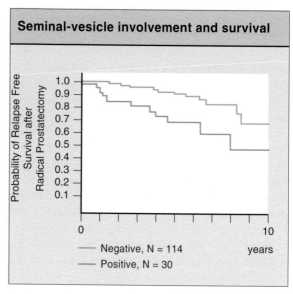

Negative, N = 114
Positive, N = 30

2.29 Seminal-vesicle involvement by prostate cancer carries a poor prognosis. (Data from Dr DF Paulson.)

Preoperative PSA vs Pathological stage (after perturbation)

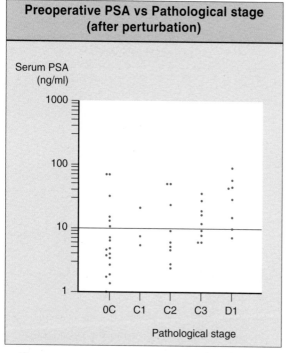

2.30 PSA and tumour stage without regard to perturbation. (Reproduced with permission from Ellis WJ, Brawer MK. Management decisions in the patient with an elevated PSA. *AUA Update Series* 1993;**XII(34)**:265–272.)

Preoperative PSA vs Pathological stage (unperturbed)

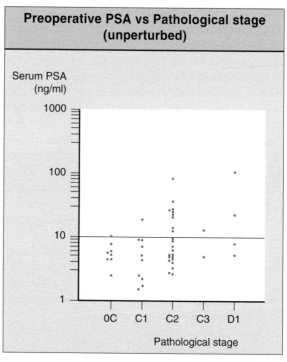

2.31 PSA and tumour stage (prebiopsy). (Reproduced with permission from Ellis WJ, Brawer MK. Management decisions in the patient with an elevated PSA. *AUA Update Series* 1993;**XII(34)**:265–272.)

4 or 5 tumour of any volume that was confined, or demonstrated microscopic extracapsular extension in cancers of any grade and any volume. Advanced neoplasms, defined as those that have extensive extracapsular extension, seminal-vesicle extension or pelvic lymph-node metastases, were not found in the cysto-prostatectomy specimens.

Of 360 men undergoing radical prostatectomy, latent carcinoma was found in 9%, curable malignancy in 62%, and in 29% of patients it was thought that advanced cancer was present and was not likely to have been cured. Among the 246 men who had palpable tumours, 8% were deemed latent, 58% curable, and 34% advanced. Of the 55% of patients who had non-palpable carcinoma (stage T1c), identified by elevation of serum PSA, 13% were felt to be latent, 76% curable, and 11% advanced.

TUMOUR VOLUME AND GLEASON GRADE

McNeal has reported that tumour volume and Gleason grade are closely correlated[37]. His data indicate that capsular penetration only begins when tumours have exceeded a volume of 0.5 cm^3, and occurs frequently when tumour volume is greater than 1.4 cm^3 (**2.28**). Oesterling[38] has also found that the Gleason grade is correlated with capsular penetration, seminal-vesicle invasion (**2.29**) and lymph-node metastases in Stage B (T2) disease. Unfortunately, at present it is often not possible to make an accurate determination of tumour volume pre-operatively. In practical terms, therefore, in patients with high-grade tumours (Gleason grade >7), additional staging procedures such as lymph-node dissection should be considered before radical

Table 2.4 Distinguishing clinically unimportant (CU) prostate cancers (N = 105, 19 CU)	
PSA and tumour volume	C.U. (%)
PSA < 4.0 ng/ml and < 1 mm	86
PSA < 4.0 and 1–5 mm	45
PSA 4-20 < 1 mm	50
PSA 4-20	14
PSA > 20 and 5 mm	0

surgery, to decrease the likelihood of operating inappropriately on patients with locally advanced or metastatic disease.

PSA AND PATHOLOGICAL STAGE

Serum prostate specific antigen (PSA) is discussed in detail in Chapter 6. Its utility as a staging tool and, by extrapolation, as a method of assessing malignant potential, was initially felt to be of low utility owing to the considerable overlap of pathological stage in patients with pre-operative PSA value. **2.30** demonstrates one initial experience, and this was reflected by the observations of many other authorities[39,40]. However, in all of these reports, care was not taken to ensure that significant prostate perturbation (which we now know can influence the serum PSA levels for a long period of time) did not contaminate these findings. In our recent radical prostatectomy series, in which preoperative PSA was obtained prior to significant prostatic perturbation (i.e. biopsy), the potential prognostic yield for elevated PSA (greater than 10.0 ng/ml) is considerable (**2.31**). Very few men with a PSA exceeding this level have lesions that can reasonably be considered to be surgically curable.

Tumour volume, as well as serum PSA, offer objective methods of assessing the malignant potential of prostate cancer. Goto and associates[41] examined 105 men and attempted to use these parameters (**Table 2.4**) to identify 19 patients with clinically insignificant cancers from those with cancer that was more likely to impact on their life.

Bluestein and associates[42] have conducted clinical studies of primary Gleason grade on biopsy and serum PSA to quantitate the risk of pelvic lymph-node metastasis in men who are subjected to a radical prostatectomy. As can be seen in **Table 2.5** for clinically localized prostate cancer, Gleason grade 1–2 and PSA less than 17.1 would afford this performance. In contrast, if the grade was Gleason 4–5, then the PSA had to be less than 4.2. These authors argued that this would mitigate against the presence of pelvic lymph-node metastasis in a high percentage of patients.

DNA PLOIDY

DNA ploidy has been extensively investigated as a prognostic marker. While several authors have felt that this modality offers significant stratification of patients' prostate cancer risk[43–45], significant problems surround this approach. O'Malley and associates[46] recently reported significant heterogeneity in the DNA ploidy. In nine radical prostatectomy specimens, they performed biopsies of the tumour and compared the DNA ploidy by flow cytometry in different aliquots. Marked ploidy differences (diploid versus tetraploid or aneuploid) were seen in five of the nine cases. Greene *et al.*[47] recently confirmed these findings by utilizing static image-analysis ploidy determinations. This degree of variability of ploidy within a given tumour markedly constrains the potential utility of this approach.

It has long been recognized[48,49] that once a neo-plasm exceeds 1 mm in diameter it has to induce a blood supply and develop an angiogenic phenotype. Weidner and associates[50] were able to stratify women with breast cancer as to the likelihood of metastasis based on the microvessel quantification. Utilizing factor VIII immunohistochemical correlations of prostate cancer, Brawer *et al.* were able to develop a computerized image-analysis system which afforded excellent correlation to manual counting of microvessels in human prostate[51]. It has recently been demonstrated that neovascularity is a good predictor of pathological

Table 2.5 Combinations of local clinical stage, primary Gleason grade and serum PSA to yield a false negative rate of 3% for positive lymph nodes

Local Clinical Stage	Primary Gleason Grade	Serum PSA (ng/ml)
T1a–T1b (A1–B1)	1 and 2 3 4 and 5	17.1 8.0 4.2
T2c (B2)	1 and 2 3 4 and 5	4.1 2.0 1.0
T3a (C1)	1 and 2 3 4 and 5	1.4 0.7 0.3

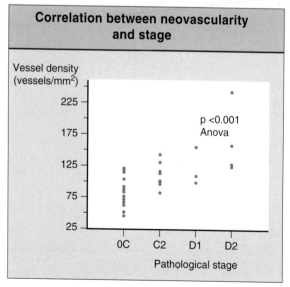

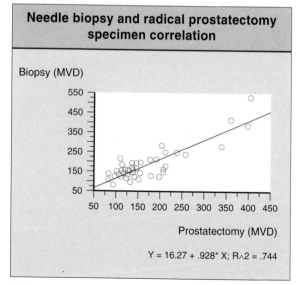

2.32 Correlation between neovascularity and tumour stage. (Modified with permission from Brawer *et al. Cancer* 1994[52].)

2.33 Microvessel density (MVD) on needle biopsy and radical prostatectomy specimen. Note strong correlation.

stage[52] (**2.32**). Moreover, it has been shown recently that in men who underwent radical prostatectomy and were shown to have pathological stage C (T_3) disease with a minimum of 10 years follow-up, neovascularity was able to stratify those patients who did not progress, whereas tumour grade was not discriminatory[51]. In addition, it has been demonstrated that there is a good correlation between microvessel density as obtained on needle biopsy, and in that found by radical prostatectomy (**2.33**). The clinical significance of neovascularity in prostate cancer has been confirmed by Weidner and associates[53] (see **4.13**).

Berges et al.[54] studied proliferation and apoptosis in normal prostate, in high-grade prostatic intra-epithelial neoplasia, and in prostatic carcinoma. They noted no difference in the percentage of proliferating cells between high-grade PIN and carcinoma, but there was more than a two-fold increase in proliferation over normal in these two conditions. What was intriguing was their observation that, when compared to normal, apoptosis, a measure of programmed cell death, was increased in high-grade PIN associated with cancer and in carcinoma itself, but was decreased in high-grade PIN not associated with cancer (**Table 2.6**).

Another important hallmark of tumour aggressiveness is its ability to invade. The prostate cancer must transgress the basement membrane to gain access to the stroma. Basement membrane has been quantified immunohistochemically using antibodies to collagen and fibronectin[55]. A strong correlation with the Gleason grade *was* observed, but these studies were hampered by the use of antibodies to type IV collagen, which could also be expressed by stromal cells. Recently, this phenomenon has been examined using antibodies to type VII collagen, which is specific to epithelial-derived basement membrane. It was demonstrated that there was a complete absence of basement membrane in carcinoma, suggesting that one of the early phenotypic changes in prostate cancer is the ability to degrade the basement membrane enzymatically.

UNUSUAL PROSTATIC TUMOURS

Adenocarcinomas arising from the epithelial lining of the secretory acini constitute by far the commonest form of malignancy of the prostate. However, other forms of tumour may occur, most of which are uncommon. These include carcinomas of other epithelial linings, such as the urethra and major prostatic ducts, as well as lymphomas, sarcomas and small-cell carcinomas. Detailed descriptions of their pathology can be found elsewhere[56] as can a discussion of their clinical manifestations[57]. Of these cancers, only a few occur with sufficient frequency to warrant description here.

Ductal Carcinomas

The glandular acini of the prostate deliver their secretions into the urethra via a complex ductal system. Tumours that arise within this system have been recognized as histologically distinct from the much more common acinar carcinomas.

Periurethral prostatic duct carcinomas have been described in detail by Kopelson et al.[58]. These carcinomas are characterized by their mixed transitional-cell/acinar morphology, and typically produce only minimal amounts of PSA.

Papillary tumours of the major prostatic ducts were originally referred to as 'endometrial' carcinomas of the prostate[59], and were thought not to be derived from prostatic duct linings. Subsequently, 'endometrial' carcinomas were shown to produce acid phosphatase[60] and PSA[61] and are now recognized as a variant of ductal carcinoma. It has been suggested, but not proven, that ductal carcinomas are more clinically aggressive than acinar tumours[62–64].

Mucinous Carcinomas

The production of mucous is not usually thought of as a characteristic of prostatic cancers, but it has been estimated that up to 20% of prostatic adenocarcinomas contain areas of mucin production[65]. However, if the suggested criterion of requiring at least 40% of the tumour demonstrating mucinous elements is applied, then the incidence of this tumour falls to less than

Table 2.6 Cell proliferation and death in the normal prostate vs. high-grade PIN and prostatic cancer (CaP)

Histology	Proliferation (%)	Apoptopic (%)
Normal	1.0	1.0
High-grade PIN	2.3 ± 0.8	0.66±0.15* 4.3 ± 0.4 **
CAP	2.2 ± 0.5	5.0 ± 0.4

*   PIN without CaP
**   PIN with CaP
(Reproduced from Berges et al. J Urol 1994[54].)

4%[66]. Fortunately, these tumours continue to secrete both acid phosphatase and PSA, and immunohistochemical stains can therefore be used to differentiate them from other mucinous carcinomas arising from either the lung or gastrointestinal tract[67] (2.27).

CONCLUSIONS

The anatomy of the prostate in the adult is largely a reflection of its embryological development. The various anatomical zones are prone to different pathological processes: BPH in the transition zone and adenocarcinoma in the peripheral zone. The underlying mechanisms for the stepwise development of these most prevalent diseases are now beginning to be unfolded by molecular biological techniques. Although detailed pathological analysis and grading can yield some insight into the aggressiveness or otherwise of prostatic tumours, more sophisticated molecular markers will be necessary to predict more precisely the metastatic potential of a cancer in a given individual. Much research is currently directed towards identifying such markers; this work, together with an insight into the molecular mechanisms of induction of prostate cancer, are the subject of the following chapters.

REFERENCES

1   Lowsley OS. The development of the human prostate gland with reference to the development of other structures of the neck of the urinary bladder. Am J Anat 1912;13:299.

2   McNeal JE. Regional morphology and pathology of the prostate. Am J Clin Pathol 1968;49:347–357.

3   Kirby RS, Lowe D, Bultitude MJ. Intraprostatic urinary reflux: an aetiological factor in abacterial prostatitis. Br J Urd 1982;54:729–731.

4   Reese JH, McNeal JE, Redwine EA, et al. Differential distribution of pepsinogen II between the zones of the human prostate and the seminal vesicle. J Urd 1986;136:1148.

5   Reese JH, McNeal JE, Redwine EA, et al. Tissue type plasminogen activator as a marker for functional zones, within the human prostate gland. Prostate 1988;12:47.

6   Villers AA, McNeal JE, Freiha FS, et al. Development of prostatic carcinoma: morphometric and pathological features of early stages. Acta Oncol 1991;30:145–149.

7   Villers A, McNeal JE, Redwine EA, Freiha FS, Stamey TA. The role of perineural space invasion in the local spread of prostatic adenocarcinoma. J Urd 1989;142:763.

8   Ayala AG, Ro JY, Babian R, Troncoso P, Grignon DJ. The prostatic capsule: does it exist? Am J Surg Pathol 1989;13:21.

9   Lepor H, Gregerman M, Crosby R, Mostofi FK, Walsh PC. Precise localization of the autonomic nerves from the pelvic plexus to the corpora cavernosa: a detailed anatomical study of the adult male pelvis. J Urd 1985;133:207–212.

10 Walsh PC, Epstein JI. Radical prostatectomy with preservation of sexual function. Impact on cancer control. Problems in Urology 1987;1(1):42–52.

11 Walsh PC, Epstein JI, Lowe FC. Potency following radical prostatectomy with wide unilateral excision of the neurovascular bundle. J Urd 1987;138:823–827.

12 Brading AF, Turner WH. The unstable bladder: towards a common mechanism. Br J Urd 1994;73:3–8.

13 Desmond PM, Clark J, Thompson IM, Zeidman EJ, Mueller EJ. Morbidity with contemporary prostate biopsy. J Urd 1993;150:1425–1426.

14 Hodge KK, McNeal SE, Terris MK, Stamey TA. Random systematic versus directed ultrasound-guided transrectal core biopsies of the prostate. J Urd 1989;142:71.

15 Ekman H, Hedberg K, Persson PS. Cytological versus histological examination of needle biopsy specimens in the diagnosis of prostatic cancer. Br J Urd 1967;39:544–548.

16 Esposti PL. Cytologic malignancy grading of prostatic carcinoma by transrectal aspiration biopsy. Scand J Urd Nephrd 1971;5:199–209.

17 Brawer MK, Bostwick DM, Peehl DM, Stamey TA. Keratin immunoreactivity in the benign and neoplastic human prostate. Canc Res 1985;45(8):3663–3667.

18 Kirby RS, Christmas TJ. Benign Prostatic Hyperplasia. London: Gower Medical Publishing, 1993; 1–109.

19 Gleason DF. Histologic grading and clinical staging of prostatic carcinoma. In: Tannenbaum M, ed. Urologic Pathology: The Prostate. Philadelphia: Lea & Febiger, 1977;171–198.

20 Epstein JI, Cho KR, Quinn BD. Relationship of severe dysplasia to Stage A (incidental) adenocarcinoma of the prostate. Cancer 1990;65:2321–2327.

21 Quinn BD, Cho KR, Epstein JI. Relationship of severe dysplasia to stage B adenocarcinoma of the prostate. Cancer 1990;65:2321–2327.

22 Bostwick DG, Brawer MK. Prostatic intraepithelial neoplasia and early invasion in prostate cancer. Cancer 1987;59:778–794.

23 Humphrey PA. Mucin in severe dysplasia in the prostate. Surg Pathol 1991;4:137–143.

24 Perlman E, Epstein JI. Blood group antigen expression in dysplasia and adenocarcinoma of the prostate. Am J Surg Pathol 1990;14:810–818.

25 McNeal JE, Alroy J, Leau I, Redwine EA, Freiha FS, Stamey TA. Immunohistochemical evidence for impaired cell differentiation in the premalignant phase of prostate carcinogenesis. Am J Clin Pathol 1988;90:23–32.

26 Nagle RB, Brewer MK, Kittelson J, Clark V. Phenotypic relationship of prostatic intraepithelial neoplasia to invasive prostatic carcinoma. Am J Pathol 1991;138:119–128.

27 Gleason DF. Histologic grading and clinical staging of prostatic carcinoma. In: Tannenbaum M, ed. *Urologic Pathology: The Prostate*. Philadelphia: Lea & Febiger, 1977.

28 Miller GJ. New developments in grading prostate cancer. *Semin Urol* 1990;**8**:9–18.

29 Gleason DF. Histologic grading of prostate cancer: a perspective. *Hum Pathol* 1992;**23**:273–279.

30 Chodak GW, Thisted RA, Gerber GS, *et al*. Results of conservative management of clinically localized prostate cancer. *New Eng J Med* 1994;**330(4)**:242–248.

31 Franks LM. Latent carcinoma of the prostate. *J Pathol Bacteriol* 1954;**68**:603–616.

32 Breslow N, Chan CW, Dhom G, *et al*. Latent carcinoma of the prostate at autopsy in seven areas. *Int J Cancer* 1977;**20**:680–688.

33 Sakr WA, Haas GP, Cassin BF, *et al*. The frequency of carcinoma of the prostate and intraepithelial neoplasia of the prostate in young male patients. *J Urol* 1993;**150**:379–385.

34 McNeal JE, Bostwick DG, Kindrachuk RA, *et al*. Patterns of progression in prostate cancer. *Lancet* 1986;**1**:60–63.

35 Scardino PT, Weaver R, Hudson MA. Early detection of prostate cancer. *Hum Pathol* 1992;**23(3)**:211.

36 Ohori M, Wheeler TM, Dunn JK,*et al*. Pathologic features and prognosis of prostate cancers detectable with current diagnostic tests. *J Urol* 1994;**151 (Suppl)**:451A No.894.

37 McNeal JE. Cancer volume and site of origin of adenocarcinoma in the prostate: relationship to local and distant spread. *Hum Pathol* 1992;**23**:258–266.

38 Oesterling JE, Brendler CB, Epstein JI, *et al*. Correlation of clinical stage, serum prostatic acid phosphatase and preoperative Gleason grade with final pathological stage in 275 patients with clinically localized adenocarcinoma of the prostate. *J Urol* 1987;**138**:92–98.

39 Oesterling JE, Chan DW, Epstein JI, *et al*. Prostate specific antigen in the preoperative and postoperative evaluation of localized prostatic cancer treated with radical prostatectomy. *J Urol* 1988;**139**:766–772.

40 Stamey TA, Yang N, Hay AR, *et al*. Prostate-specific antigen as a serum marker for adenocarcimoma of the prostate. *New Eng J Med* 1987;**317**:909–916.

41 Goto Y, Ohori M, Arakawa A, Wheeler TM, Scardino PT. Distinguishing clinically important from unimportant prostate cancers before treatment: preliminary report. *J Urol* 1994;**151(Suppl)**:289A No.248.

42 Bluestein DL, Bostwick DG, Bergstralb EJ, *et al*. Eliminating the need for bilateral pelvic lymphadenectomy in select patients with prostate cancer. *J Urol* 1994;**151**:1315–1320.

43 Lee SE, Currin SM, Paulson DF, *et al*. Flow cytometric determination of ploidy in prostatic adenocarcinoma: A comparison with seminal vesicle involvement and histopathologic grading as a predictor of clinical recurrence. *J Urol* 1988;**140**:769–774.

44 Stephenson RA, James BCHG, Fair WR, *et al*. Flow cytometry of prostate cancer: Relationship of DNA content to survival. *Canc Res* 1987;**47**:2504–2507.

45 Zetterberg A, Eposti PL. Prostatic significance of nuclear DNA levels in prostatic carcinoma. *Scand J Urol Nephrol* 1980;**55**:53–56.

46 O'Malley FP, Grignon DJ, Keeney M,*et al*. DNA heterogeneity in prostatic adenocarcinoma: A DNA flow cytometric mapping study with whole organ section of prostate. *Cancer* 1993;**71(9)**:2797.

47 Greene DR, Taylor SR, Wheeler TM *et al*. DNA ploidy by image analysis of individual foci of prostate cancer: A preliminary report. *Canc Res* 1991;**51**:4084.

48 Folkman J, Cole P, Zimmerman S. Tumour behaviour in isolated perfused organs: in vitro growth and metastasis of biopsy material in rabbit thyroid and canine intestinal segment. *Ann Surg* 1966;**164**:491.

49 Folkman J. Tumour angiogenesis: therapeutic implications. *N Engl J Med* 1971;**285**:1182.

50 Weidner N, Semple J, Welch W, *et al*. Tumor angiogenesis and metastasis – correlation in invasive breast carcinoma. *New Eng J Med* 1971;**285**:1182.

51 Brawer MK, Jonsson E, Gibbons RP, *et al*. Extent of prostate neovascularity predicts progression in patients with pathologic stage C adenocarcinoma treated with radical prostatectomy. *J Urol* 1994;**151(Suppl)**:289A' No.246.

52 Brawer MK, Deering RE, Brown M, *et al*. Predictors of pathologic stage in prostatic carcinoma. The role of neovascularity. *Cancer* 1994;**73(3)**:678–687.

53 Weidner N, Carrol PR, Flax J, *et al*. Tumour angiogenesis correlates with metastasis in invasive prostate carcinoma. *Am J Pathol* 1993;**143(2)**:401–409.

54 Berges R, Carmichael M, Epstein JI, *et al*. Cell proliferation and death in the normal prostate vs. high grade PIN and prostatic cancer. *J Urol* 1994;**151 (Suppl)**:No.196.

55 Fuchs MF, Brawer MK, Rennels MA, *et al*. The relationship of basement membrane to histologic grade of human prostatic carcinoma. *Modern Path* 1989;**2(2)**:105–111.

56 Miller GJ. An atlas of prostatic biopsies: dilemmas of morphologic variance. In: Fenoglio-Preiser CM, Wolff M, Rilke F, eds. *Progress in Surgical Pathology* VIII. Philadelphia: Field and Wood, 1988;81–112.

57 Efros MD, Fischer J, Mallouh C, *et al*. Unusual primary prostatic malignancies. *Urology* 1992;**39**:407–410.

58 Kopelson G, Harisiadis L, Romos NA, *et al*. Periurethral prostatic duct carcinoma: clinical features and treatment results. *Cancer* 1978;**42**:2894–2902.

59 Melicow MM, Pachter MR. Endometrial carcinoma of prostatic utricle (uterus masculinus). *Cancer* 1967;**20**:1715–1722.

60 Nadji M, Tabei SZ, Castro A, *et al*. Prostatic origin of tumours: an immunohistochemical study. *Am J Clin Pathol* 1980;**73**:735–739.

61 Walker AN, Mills SE, Fechner RE, *et al*. 'Endometrial' adeno-carcinoma of the prostatic urethra arising in a villous polyp: a light microscopic and immunoperoxidase study. *Arch Pathol Lab Med* 1982;**106**:624–627.

62 Dube VE, Farrow GM, Greene LF. Prostatic adenocarcinoma of ductal origin. *Cancer* 1973;**32**:402–409.

63 Greene LF, Farrow GM, Ravits JM, *et al*. Prostatic adeno-carcinoma of duct origin. *J Urol* 1979;**121**:303–305.

64 Lemberger RJ, Bishop MC, Bates CP, *et al*. Carcinoma of the prostate of ductal origin. *Br J Urol* 1984;**56**:706–709.

65 Elbadawi A, Craig W, Linke CA, *et al*. Prostatic mucinous carcinoma. *Urology* 1979;**13**:658–666.

66 Epstein JI, Lieberman PH. Mucinous adenocarcinoma of the prostate gland. *Am J Surg Pathol* 1985;**9**:299–308.

67 Odom DG, Donatucci CF, Deshon GE. Mucinous adenocarcinoma of the prostate. *Hum Pathol* 1990;**21**:593–600.

CHAPTER 3

EPIDEMIOLOGY AND NATURAL HISTORY OF PROSTATE CANCER

INTRODUCTION

Although prostate cancer seems set to become the most common malignant disease to affect males in both the developed and developing world, the high prevalence of other concurrent diseases that can also be fatal in elderly males means that this neoplasm is not always the primary cause of death. As most patients with prostate cancer are beyond middle age, the average number of life-years lost – around 9 – is lower than that for other tumours (**Table 3.1**). However, since the disease is so common, the *cumulative* potential years of life lost make it third among all cancers (**Table 3.2**). Also, as noted in the previous chapter, although the prevalence of clinical prostate cancer is very high, it has become apparent that there are far larger numbers of males who have a so-called

'latent', well-differentiated microscopic form of the disease that may never progress to invasive clinical disease with metastatic potential; the natural history of these 'incidental' cancers is currently not well understood.

INCIDENCE

It is difficult to estimate the worldwide prevalence of clinical prostate cancer due to insufficient data from developing countries. Of course, the shorter life-expectancy in these countries means that prostate cancer is less likely to be a clinical problem or cause of death. The most complete epidemiological data derive mainly from the USA, where the incidence of clinical prostate cancer has been fairly accurately documented. In the USA, the incidence of newly diagnosed cases of prostate cancer was 100 000

Table 3.1 Average life-years lost by premature death from several cancers in the USA			
	Prostate (men)	Breast (women)	Lung (both sexes)
Average years of life lost	9.0	19.2	13.5(men) 14.8(women)
(Modified with permission from Montie JE *Urology* 1994;**44**(6A):2–8.)			

Table 3.2 Potential life-years lost by premature death from several cancers in the USA			
	Prostate (men)	Breast (women)	Lung (both sexes)
Potential years of life lost	228 547	763 511	2 870 113
(Modified with permission from Montie JE *Urology* 1994;**44**(6A):2–8.)			

Table 3.3 Deaths in 1990 from several cancers in individuals under age 75 years

Cancer	Deaths
Prostate	12 423
Lung	100 253
Breast	29 931
Colon/rectum	29 805

Table 3.4 Predisposing factors for clinical prostate cancer

Genetic	Familial autosomal dominant in some
Racial	Commoner in blacks, Scandinavians, US whites and Western Europeans
Age	Commoner with increasing age
Hormones	Testosterone and dihydro-testosterone apparently essential
Sexual history	Commoner in men with early sexual experience and multiple sexual partners
Diet	Animal fats
	Low intake of yellow/green vegetables
Pollution	Urban dwelling
	Cadmium exposure
	Exposure to radioactive agents: Tritium, ^{51}Cr, ^{59}Fe, ^{60}Co, ^{65}Zn
Infection	Gonococcal infection?
	Herpes simplex type 2?
	RNA viruses?
Vasectomy	Increases risk?

? = possible risk factors

in 1988, and this had risen incrementally to 132 000 in 1992[1]; the projected incidence for 1994 was only a little less than 200 000 (**3.1**). Although this rise in new cases of prostate cancer may result, at least in part, from an increased awareness of and search for the condition by screening programmes utilizing PSA, it is becoming clear that clinically significant prostate cancer is also on the increase. Autopsy studies have identified foci of prostate cancer in approximately 20% of men in their 20s, 30% of men in their 50s and 70% of the over 80s[2]. However, as mentioned, the lifetime chance of a man developing clinically apparent prostate cancer is less than 10%[3]; hence, the large majority of the small prostate cancers detected at autopsy are clinically insignificant, or 'latent' cancers. Although the majority of these tiny, well-differentiated prostate cancers apparently grow only very slowly within the natural lifespan of the individual, a proportion de-differentiate, grow rapidly and metastasize, leading to a fatal outcome. Mortality attributable to prostate cancer was 28 000 in the USA in 1988 and has risen steadily since then to around 36 000 in 1994 (**3.2**). A similar time trend in both incidence and mortality of prostate cancer is also apparent in the UK (**3.3**). The rise in incidence and mortality attributable to prostate cancer in the Netherlands

Table 3.5 Protective factors for clinical prostate cancer

Racial	Rare in Asians
Age	Rare in young men
Hormones	Absent in pseudo-hermaphrodites and eunuchs
Diet	High intake of yellow/green vegetables
	Low fat intake, especially red meat
Environment	Less common in rural dwellings
Hepatic cirrhosis	Due to increased oestrogen

has been shown to be due to a 'birth-cohort' effect in which males born in consecutive years have an increasing risk of developing prostate cancer[4]. This increase in prostate cancer-related death is more than one would expect from demographic changes in the age of the population alone, and has occurred in the United States in spite of relatively active treatment of localized disease by radiation and radical prostatectomy.

Clinically significant prostate cancer is rare in men under the age of 50 years. As with latent prostate cancer, however, the incidence increases more rapidly with age than that of any other tumour. In addition to this, the mortality attributable to prostate cancer increases steadily with increasing age from 50 years upwards (**3.4**). However, many of those dying are younger than 75 years of age (**Table 3.3**).

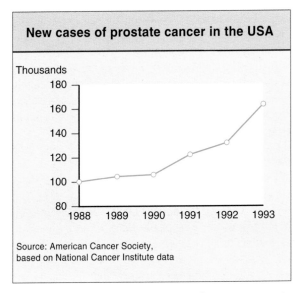

Source: American Cancer Society, based on National Cancer Institute data

3.1 Rising incidence of newly diagnosed prostate cancer in the USA.

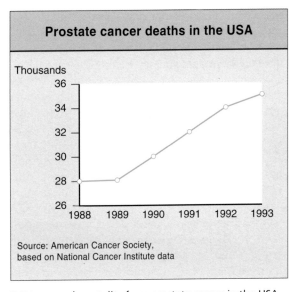

Source: American Cancer Society, based on National Cancer Institute data

3.2 Increased mortality from prostate cancer in the USA.

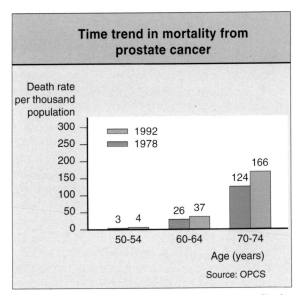

Source: OPCS

3.3 Time trend in increased prostate cancer mortality by age in England and Wales, 1978 and 1992.

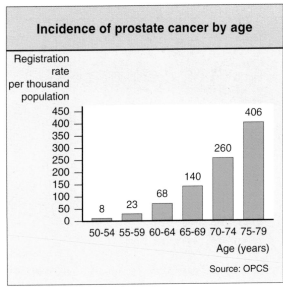

Source: OPCS

3.4 Mortality from prostate cancer in England and Wales by age cohort, 1987.

Familial Prostate Cancer

It has recently become apparent that there is a greater-than-expected incidence of prostate cancer in the male relatives of men who have died from the disease. A study of 228 men dying of prostate cancer revealed a relative risk of prostate cancer in fathers and siblings that was nearly three times higher than that of a control group[5]. A genealogical study of cancer in Mormons living in Utah examined the occurrence of 2 821 cases of prostate cancer occurring between 1958 and 1961. This demonstrated that prostate cancer had the fourth highest familial association of all cancers studied, with a stronger familial link than both colonic and breast cancer, which are generally regarded as having a significant genetic component[6]. A study of 691 men with prostate cancer revealed twice the expected incidence of prostate cancer in those with first-degree relatives with the disease. Also, those men with two or three affected first-degree relatives had a 5-fold and 11-fold increased lifetime risk of developing prostate cancer respectively[7]. Currently, about 9% of all cases of prostatic cancer are thought to have a genetic basis – this is about twice the percentage of the familial tumours seen in breast cancer.

Clearly the increased incidence of prostate cancer among members of the same family could result from environmental factors rather than a genetic predisposition. Recently, however, some evidence has emerged to suggest that a genuinely hereditary form of prostate cancer may exist. Hereditary prostate cancer is characterized by Mendelian autosomal dominant inheritance, and an early onset of the disease[8]. At the time of writing, the location and determinants of the gene or genes that might be responsible for hereditary prostate cancer have not been elucidated, but loss of one or more tumour suppressor gene loci seems the most likely explanation (see Chapter 4).

Mass screening by specific invitation of asymptomatic men for prostate cancer is at present controversial (see Chapter 7). However, there is now strong evidence to support the value of screening of first-degree male relatives of men with prostate cancer, particularly male relatives of those developing the disease at a young age and those with a strong positive family history of the disease. Since congenital prostate cancer has an early onset, this screening process should start around the age of 40.

Geographical and Ethnic Variations

The worldwide prevalence of clinical prostate cancer varies remarkably from one country to another. The highest reported incidence is from the Scandinavian countries (60 per 100 000 per year), with intermediate incidence in the USA (50 per 100 000) and the UK (20 per 100 000). The lowest incidence is in the Far East, especially in mainland China and Japan (4 per 100 000). The difference between the highest and lowest is almost 100 fold. Unfortunately, accurate figures are not available from many countries of the world, although high-risk, medium-risk and low-risk zones can be identified (3.5).

The rate of mortality attributable to prostate cancer is also highly variable worldwide. The highest rate of mortality from prostate cancer occurs in the West Indies and Bermuda, at 28–29 per 100 000. The mortality rates from the USA and the UK are 15 per 100 000 and 12 per 100 000 respectively. It is interesting to note the disparity between the incidence:mortality ratio between the USA and the UK: 50:20 per 100 000 and 15:12 per 100 000 respectively. It has been suggested that this might result from aggressive therapy for early disease in the form of radical prostatectomy that is common practice in the USA, but less commonly performed in the UK. However, in the USA, the death rate from prostate cancer has increased together with the incidence rates, in spite of an increase in the number of radical prostatectomies performed. It is therefore

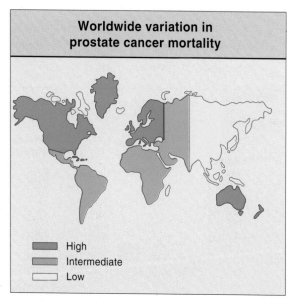

Worldwide variation in prostate cancer mortality

High
Intermediate
Low

3.5 Geographical distribution of high-risk, medium-risk and low-risk areas for prostate cancer.

possible that the increasing incidence of prostate cancer in the USA, over and above that seen in the UK, to some extent reflects an increase in the early diagnosis by PSA driven screening programmes. This raises the question of whether at least a proportion of the early prostate cancers diagnosed in the USA may be 'incidental' cancers that might not progress to clinically significant disease if left untreated. This issue will be further addressed in subsequent chapters.

Further analysis of the statistics for the incidence of prostate cancer in multiracial communities has shown wide differences between races. The highest incidence is found in blacks, and the lowest in Chinese and Japanese races. This finding also explains, at least in part, the enormous geographical variation in the incidence of prostate cancer. The highest worldwide incidence of prostate cancer is in blacks living in Atlanta, Georgia (91.2 per 100 000), while the lowest is in Chinese residents of Shanghai (1.3 per 100 000). However, blacks living in Africa appear to have a lower rate of prostate cancer, although this may simply result from the shorter life expectancy in Africa and the limited facilities for diagnosis. Epidemiological data have also shown a disparity between the incidence of prostate cancer in racial groups in their native countries and migrants of the same group living in countries with a higher endemic rate of prostate cancer. In particular, Japanese migrants to the Bay area of San Francisco have an incidence of prostate cancer of 16.5 per 100 000, whilst their counterparts remaining in Osaka, Japan, have an incidence of only 6.1 per 100 000). A similar difference has been described in Japanese migrants to Hawaii[9]. However, the incidence of prostate cancer in such Japanese migrants does not rise anywhere near as high as that for endemic whites in San Francisco (50 per 100 000). Similar differences are found in migrant Chinese, Jews and Indians. It is interesting to note that the incidence of latent or incidental prostate cancer appears to affect all groups equally. These data suggest an in-born genetic predisposition for the development of prostate cancer associated with specific racial groups, with superadded promotion of disease progression by environmental factors.

AETIOLOGICAL AND PREDISPOSING FACTORS FOR PROSTATE CANCER

Apart from the 9% or so of men with hereditary prostate cancer, the strongest predetermining factor for the development of prostate cancer is age. As already mentioned, prostate cancer is rarely found in the under 50s but is increasingly common with rising age (**3.4**). The racial characteristics outlined above are also quite strong predisposing factors with North American blacks, having roughly twice the lifetime risk of the disease compared with their white counterparts.

Hormones

Circulating androgens are an essential prerequisite for the growth of normal prostate, and for the development of benign prostatic hyperplasia and prostate-cancer change. The precise role of androgens in terms of carcinogenesis within the prostate is not entirely clear, but they seem to act by promoting cell growth and division. Although the amount of circulating testosterone is variable from one individual to another, there is apparently no direct correlation between the serum testosterone level and the risk of developing prostate cancer[10]. It is interesting to note that although serum testosterone levels gradually decline with advancing age, the incidence of prostate cancer steadily increases. This apparent anomaly might be explained by the lengthy lag period between initial early neoplastic change and the appearance of clinically apparent prostate cancer, as well as by changes in androgen receptor levels.

Testosterone is metabolized within the prostate to dihydrotestosterone (DHT) by the enzyme 5-alpha reductase. It is now known that it is DHT rather than testosterone which is the major intracellular androgen that promotes growth within the prostate[11]. The role of DHT in the promotion of prostate cancer is as yet unclear. However, prostate cancer does not appear to occur in a cohort of pseudohermaphrodite men in whom 5-alpha reductase is absent. It is also possible that the variable geographical incidence of prostate cancer might be related in some way to different levels of DHT in ethnic groups. In particular a reduced activity of 5-alpha reductase has been reported in Japanese men – this could perhaps account for the lower, but currently rising, prevalence of prostate cancer in Japan[12].

Cirrhosis of the liver can lead to a decrease in the level of circulating testosterone as well as an increase in circulating oestrogens; both of these changes could account for the reduced risk of developing prostate cancer in this condition[13].

The precise role of androgens in the induction and promotion or progression of prostate cancer is not yet fully understood. However, once malignant transformation has become established, androgens almost certainly have a role in stimulating malignant cell activity and division.

Diet

There has been considerable interest in the role of dietary components in the aetiology of prostate cancer. The high incidence of prostate cancer in the USA appears to correlate with an increase in fat consumption. Regions within the USA where dairy product and red-meat ingestion is greatest also have a higher age-adjusted incidence of prostate cancer[14].

There are several potential modes of action of fats in prostate cancer. In some strains of genetically susceptible rats, certain fats reduce the induction time for testosterone to stimulate the development of prostate cancer[15]. Another possible mechanism whereby high levels of fat consumption increase the risk of prostate cancer is reduction in the absorption of vitamin A. An increase in the circulating level of beta-carotene, which depends upon the amount of vitamin A absorption, appears to be protective against the development of some cancers[16]. Circulating testosterone levels decrease by as much as 30% in men converted to a vegetarian low-fat diet, and could hence reduce the induction of prostate cancer by testosterone[17]. In Japan, where the traditional diet is low in fat, the incidence of prostate cancer has recently begun to rise in association with increasing 'Westernization' of lifestyle. Similar trends seem to be occurring in China[18].

The traditional diets in Japan and other Asian countries consist of large quantities of yellow and green vegetables. High levels of vitamin A in this diet may protect against the induction of prostate cancer. Also, phyto-oestrogens found in vegetables such as soya may alter the hormonal milieu and counteract the effects of testerone upon the prostate, hence reducing the incidence of prostate cancer.

The substantial worldwide variation in the incidence of prostate cancer appears to depend to some extent upon genetic factors, but dietary differences could account for the changes in incidence in migration studies. It seems likely that the Western diet, which is high in animal fats and relatively low in vegetables, confers a higher risk for the development of prostate cancer.

Sexual Activity

It has been suggested that frequent sexual activity initiated early in life, multiple sexual partners and a history of sexually transmitted diseases may all increase the risk of prostate cancer[19]. Correlation between a history of gonococcal infection and prostate cancer, with a 45-year delay period, has been reported[20]. However, there are also conflicting data suggesting an increase in prostate cancer in men with low levels of sexual activity[21], and a study has shown that prostate cancer mortality in 1400 reputedly celibate Catholic priests was comparable to that within the general male population[22]. At present, the influence of sexual activity on the development of prostate cancer should be considered uncertain, but the changes in sexual mores occurring since the 1960s may well manifest themselves in a greater prevalence of prostate cancer in years to come. The median age at first intercourse for men in the UK, for example, has fallen from 20 to 17 over the last 25 years. The number of sexual partners during the lifetime of the average man has also increased considerably[23].

Vasectomy

Considerable controversy has surrounded a study suggesting a causal link between vasectomy and the subsequent development of prostate cancer[24]. However, this case-control surveillance can be criticized since it was not a prospective analysis, did not take account of other potential variable influences (such as sexual history and testosterone level) and did not exclude the presence of occult cancer in case controls. Two recent studies by Giovannucci[25,26] suggested a relative risk for vasectomy patients for prostate cancer of 1.85 and 1.56. Other studies of larger numbers of men who had undergone vasectomy failed to demonstrate conclusively an increased risk of prostate cancer[27]. At present, there seems no good reason to counsel against this important method of limiting world population growth, although individuals contemplating this procedure should probably be advised that the question remains open[28].

Environmental Factors

Over the last few decades, attention has increasingly been focused on the possible role of environmental pollution in promoting a number of neoplastic diseases. Exposure to a variety of chemicals that have been widely used in industry has been shown to contribute towards the development of particular malignant tumours. Prostate cancer is less likely to develop in men living in a rural environment than in their counterparts living within cities, and the latter group are also at greater risk of dying from the disease[14]. The factor, or factors, responsible for this could be general environmental pollution by chemical agents, as well as exposure to substances within the work place. Workers exposed to chemicals in the rubber, textile, chemical, drug, fertilizer and atomic energy industries have an increased risk of developing prostate cancer. The precise chemicals responsible for inducing prostate cancer are not known, although the finding of increased levels of cadmium in patients with prostate cancer has led to the suggestion that this might induce the condition[29]. There is also evidence to suggest that exposure to tritium, ^{51}Cr, ^{59}Fe, ^{60}Co, and ^{65}Zn may increase the risk of prostate cancer in employees of the United Kingdom Atomic Energy Authority[30]. Car salesmen, caretakers, personnel managers and shipping clerks have also been suggested to be at increased risk of developing prostate cancer. It is difficult to explain these associations (at least in terms of chemical exposure), and it seems likely that there are many other, as yet unknown, environmental factors associated with twentieth century living that might act to promote small foci of incidental prostate cancer to become locally invasive.

Smoking

Although tobacco smoking has been implicated as an aetiological factor in malignant tumours of the lung and bladder and many other neoplasms, no such association has yet been found in prostate cancer[31].

Viruses

Infectious agents, particularly viruses, are known to be the cause of carcinogenesis in some forms of genital malignancy such as cervical cancer. Viruses are certainly a potential environmental trigger for prostate cancer, but this is difficult to prove since many viruses are ubiquitous and others are impossible to isolate from tumour cells.

A possible candidate for the aetiology of prostate cancer is herpes simplex virus type 2. Antibodies to this virus were detected within the serum of 71% of prostate cancer cases, but in only 66% of controls with benign prostatic hyperplasia[32]. The virus has also been demonstrated within prostate cancer cells by electron microscopy[33]. It is intruiging to note also that wives of men with prostate cancer were reported to have an increased incidence of cervical carcinoma in one study[34].

RNA viral particles have also been identified within prostate cancer cells[35]. Further support for an aetio-logical role for RNA viruses is the presence of the H-ras oncogene p21 within prostate cancer cells. This seems to be associated with less well-differentiated prostate cancers[36].

PROSTATE CANCER AND BENIGN PROSTATIC HYPERPLASIA

The possibility of a causal association between prostate cancer and benign prostatic hyperplasia (BPH) is still controversial. Prostate cancer most commonly arises within the peripheral part of the prostate, while BPH predominantly develops within the transition zone[37]. However, Armenian et al.[38] reported that patients with BPH have a risk of developing prostate cancer that is several times greater than that of men without BPH. It was also suggested that prostatectomy reduces the chance of the subsequent development of prostate cancer. This study, however, can be criticized since the diagnosis of BPH in some of the cases was made on clinical rather than precise histological grounds.

A conflicting conclusion was reached by Greenwald and colleagues in a prospective study of men undergoing sub-total prostatectomy and a control group. The relative risk for the development of prostate cancer in the BPH group was found to be 0.88[39].

Both BPH and prostate cancer are very common in elderly males, and both are neoplastic conditions characterized by disturbances of the control of growth of prostatic epithelium. As will be discussed in the next chapter, the stepwise accumulation of genetic changes could underlie the pathogenesis of both conditions, although it currently seems unlikely that BPH is a direct precursor of adenocarcinoma.

NATURAL HISTORY OF PROSTATE CANCER

Attempts to study the natural history of prostate cancer have often been confounded by the addition of surgical, radiotherapeutic and endocrine therapies, which undoubtedly alter the long-term outcome of the disease. In the majority of circumstances, ethical and humanitarian reasons usually make it impossible to observe the natural course of this malignant disease without therapeutic intervention. However, a recent, pooled multicentre analysis of 828 men with clinically localized prostate cancer that was treated conservatively has revealed a disease-specific 10-year survival of 94% for men with a well-differentiated tumour. By contrast, there was only a 58% 10-year survival for men with a less well-differentiated tumour[40] (**3.6**).

This, and other studies, have supported the concept that some well-differentiated prostate cancers may not require active treatment, especially in older patients. Any therapeutic intervention, radical prostatectomy, radiotherapy or endocrine treatment, it has been argued, may be of no greater benefit than watchful waiting in such cases. Small foci of well-differentiated prostate cancer appear much earlier than had previously been appreciated. Recent autopsy studies have demonstrated small foci of intra-epithelial neoplasia and adenocarcinoma within the prostate in men in their 20s[41]. It seems, therefore, that the natural history of prostate cancer in at least some individuals is much more prolonged than had been appreciated.

There are probably three important steps in the natural history of prostate cancer. First, the development of microfoci of 'incidental' prostate cancer. Second, the progression from occult to clinically significant localized prostate cancer and, third, metastasis of the cancer to lymph nodes, bones or other organs. The factors influencing each of these steps are discussed in the next chapter. There are two basic explanations for the progression of prostate cancer from occult disease to clinically significant disease. The first, championed by Stamey, suggests that the development of prostate cancer is a slow but unrelenting progression. The doubling time for prostate cancer has been shown to be much slower than in other tumours (up to 4 years in some cases) so that the progression time from initial malignant transformation until the appearance of a 1 ml volume tumour may be as long as 10 years[42]. The second consideration is that multiple genetic hits are necessary for transformation into clinically significant prostate cancer and subsequent dedifferentiation, and that in some men occult prostate cancer will never progress. This could also explain the fact that, although the prevalence of histological prostate cancer is evenly distributed worldwide, clinical disease develops to a variable extent in different countries dependent upon environmental factors[43] that act as promoters of progression. These issues are considered in greater depth in the next chapter.

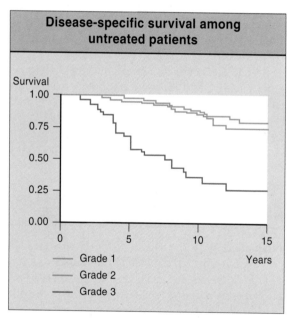

3.6 Disease-specific survival among untreated patients with prostate cancer according to tumour grade (modified from Chodak *et al. NEJM* 1994 **330**: 242–248).

REFERENCES

1 Boring CC, Squires TS, Tong T. Cancer statistics 1993. CA *Cancer Clin J* 1993;**43**:7–26.
2 Sheldon CA, Williams RD, Fraley EE. Incidental carcinoma of the prostate; a review of the literature and critical reappraisal of classification. J *Urol* 1980;**124**:626–631.
3 Silverberg E, Lubera JA. Cancer statistics. CA 1989;**39**:3–20.
4 van der Gulden JWJ, Kiemeney LALM, Verbeek ALM, *et al.* Mortality trend from prostate cancer in the Netherlands (1950–1989). *Prostate* 1994;**24**:33–38.
5 Woolf CM. An investigation of the familial aspects of carcinoma of the prostate. *Cancer* 1960;**13**:739–743.
6 Cannon L, Bishop DT, Skolnick M, *et al.* Genetic epidemiology of prostate cancer in the Utah Mormon genealogy. *Cancer Survey* 1982;**1**:47.
7 Steinberg GS, Carter BS, Beaty TH, *et al.* Family history and the risk of prostate cancer. *Prostate* 1990;**17**:337–340.
8 Carter BS, Beaty TH, Steinberg GD, *et al.* Mendelian inheritance of familial prostate cancer. *Proceedings of the National Academy of Science* 1992;**89**:3367–3370.
9 Akazaki K, Stemmermann GN. Comparative study of latent carcinoma of the prostate among Japanese in Japan and Hawaii. JNCI, 1973;**50**:1137.
10 Ghanadian R, Pugh CM, O'Donoghue EPN. Serum testosterone and dihydrotestosterone in carcinoma of the prostate. British *Journal of Cancer* 1979;**9**:696.
11 Bruchovsky N, Wilson JD The conversion of testosterone to 5-alpha-androstan-17-beta-ol-3-one by rat prostate *in vivo* and *in vitro. Journal of Biological Chemistry* 1968;**243**: 2012–2021.

12 Ross RK, Bernstein L, Loba RA *et al.* 5-alpha-reductase activity and risk of prostate cancer among Japanese and US white and black males. *Lancet* 1992;**9**:887–889.

13 Glantz GM. Cirrhosis and carcinoma of the prostate gland. *J Urol* 1964;**91**:291.

14 Blair A, Fraumeni JF. Geographic patterns of prostate cancer in the United States. *J National Cancer Institute*, 1978;**61**:1379.

15 Pollard M, Luckert PH. Promotional effects of testosterone and dietary fat on prostate carcinogenesis in genetically susceptible rats. *Prostate* 1985;**6**:1.

16 Peto R, Doll R, Buckley JD *et al.* Can beta-carotene materially reduce human cancer rates? *Nature* 1981;**290**:201.

17 Hill PB, Wynder EL. Effect of a vegetarian diet and dexamethasone on plasma prolactin, testosterone and dehydroepiandrosterone in men and women. *Cancer Letters* 1979;**7**:273–282.

18 Gu FL, Xia TL, Kong XT. Preliminary study of the frequency of benign prostatic hyperplasia and prostatic cancer in China. *Urology* 1994;**44**:688–691.

19 Steele R, Lees RE, Kraus AJ, *et al.* Sexual factors in the epidemiology of cancer of the prostate. *Journal of Chronic Diseases* 1971;**24**:29–37.

20 Heshmat MY, Kovi J, Herson J. Epidemiologic association between gonorrhoea and prostatic carcinoma. *Urology* 1975;**6**:457.

21 Rotkin ID. Studies in the epidemiology of prostate cancer: expanded sampling. *Cancer Treatment Rep* 1977;**61**:173.

22 Ross RK, Deapen D, Casagrade J, *et al.* A cohort study of mortality from cancer of the prostate in Catholic priests. *British Journal of Cancer* 1981;**43**:223–235.

23 Editorial. Sex education in schools: peers to the rescue? *Lancet* 1994;**344**:899–900.

24 Rosenberg L, Palmer JR, Zauber AG, *et al.* Vasectomy and the risk of prostate cancer. *Am J Epidemiology* 1990;**132**:1051–1055.

25 Giovannucci E, Tosteson D, Speizer FE, *et al.* A retrospective cohort study of vasectomy and prostate cancer in US men. *JAMA* 1993;**269**:878–914.

26 Giovannucci E, Ascherio A, Rimm EB, *et al.* A prospective cohort study of vasectomy and prostate cancer in US men. *JAMA* 1993;**269**:873–877.

27 Sidney S. Vasectomy and the risk of prostate cancer and benign prostatic hypertrophy. *J Urol* 1987;**138**:795–797.

28 Howards SS, Peterson HB. Vasectomy and prostate cancer, chance bias, or a causal relationship? *JAMA* 1993;**269**:913–914.

29 Kipling MD, Waterhouse JAH. Cadmium and prostatic carcinoma. *Lancet* 1967;**1**:730.

30 Rooney C, Beral V, Maconochie N, *et al.* Case-control study of prostate cancer in employees of the United Kingdom Atomic Energy Authority. *BMJ* 1993;**307**:1391–1397.

31 Wynder EL, Mabuchi K, Whitmore WF. Epidemiology of cancer of the prostate. *Cancer* 1971;**28**:344–360.

32 Herbert JT, Birkhoff JD, Feorino PM, *et al.* Herpes simplex virus type 2 and cancer of the prostate. *J. Urol* 1976;**116**:1608–1611.

33 Centifano YM, Kaufman HE, Zam ZS *et al.* Herpes virus particles in prostate cancer cells. *J Virol* 1973;**12**:1608.

34 Feminella JJ, Lattimer JK. An apparent increase in genital carcinomas among wives of men with prostatic carcinoma: an epidemiologic survey. *Pirquet Bulletin of Clinical Medicine* 1974;**20**:3–9.

35 McCombs RM. Role of oncornaviruses in carcinoma of the prostate. *Cancer Treatment Rep* 1977;**61**:131.

36 Viola MV, Fromowitz F, Oravez S *et al.* Expression of ras oncogene p21 in prostate cancer. *New Eng J Med* 1986;**314**:133–136.

37 Breslow N, Chan CE, Dhom G, *et al.* Latent carcinoma of the prostate at autopsy in seven areas. *International Journal of Cancer* 1977;**20**:680–688.

38 Armenian NK, Lilienfeld AM, Diamond EL, *et al.* Relation between benign prostatic hyperplasia and cancer of the prostate: a prospective and retrospective study. *Lancet* 1974;**2**:115–117.

39 Greenwald P, Kirmss V, Polan AK, *et al.* Cancer of the prostate among men with benign prostatic hyperplasia. *Journal of the National Cancer Institute* 1974;**5**:35–40.

40 Chodak GW, Thisted RA, Gerber GS, *et al.* Results of conservative management of clinically localised prostate cancer. *New Eng J Med* 1994;**330**:242–248.

41 Sakr WA, Haas GP, Cassin BF, *et al.* The frequency of carcinoma and intra-epithelial neoplasia of the prostate in young male patients. *J Urol* 1993;**150**:379–385.

42 Stamey TA. Cancer of the prostate: An analysis of some important contributions and dilemmas. *Monographs in Urology* 1982;**3**:67–74.

43 Carter HB, Piantadosi S, Isaacs JT. Clinical evidence for and implications of the multistep development of prostate cancer. *J Urol* 1990;**143**:742–746.

CHAPTER 4

THE MOLECULAR BASIS OF PROSTATE CANCER

The molecular basis of prostate cancer has remained enigmatic for decades. However, progress has been made in leaps and bounds recently due to the exponential growth in our understanding of cell biology that has stemmed from recombinant DNA technology. Perhaps because prostate cancer is a disease affecting men mainly beyond middle-age, it has received only a fraction of the research endeavour dedicated to other common forms of cancer such as that of the colon or lung. This situation is at last changing; more funds are being devoted to the study of a disease that is perceived as an ever-increasing menace. Moreover, much of the new information gained about the basic science of other cancers (such as cancer of the colon and hormone-dependent breast cancer) is also applicable to malignant disease of the prostate.

HORMONAL INFLUENCES ON PROSTATE GROWTH

The normal prostate, although present structurally from around the 12th week of intrauterine life, remains rudimentary throughout childhood and develops only after puberty under the influence of increased levels of circulating androgens. Testosterone (T) is the hormone that is mainly responsible, and is synthesized by the Leydig cells of the testis under the influence of luteinizing hormone (LH) of pituitary origin. The secretion of this decapeptide is itself regulated by luteinizing-hormone releasing hormone (LHRH) from the hypothalamus. It is at this location that testosterone has a negative feedback effect which enables levels of circulating testosterone to be maintained within the normal limits (10–35 µg/l). Diurnal variation in testosterone levels (within this range) is usual, with peak plasma concentrations being recorded in the early mornings. Ninety five percent of circulating testosterone is bound to a number of plasma proteins, the predominant form of which is sex-hormone binding globulin (SHBG). This leaves only a small proportion

of the residual free androgen to enter cells by simple diffusion.

A further, much smaller source of androgens is the adrenal cortex. Under the influence of ACTH, androstene and androstenedione are released into the circulation from the adrenal glands. When testicular function is intact, this minor additional androgen activity has little impact; after chemical or physical castration, however, their residual androgenic effect may result in the survival of some clones of androgen-dependent cancer cells, possibly to the detriment of the patient[1] (**4.1**).

Androgen stimulation of prostate cancer cells

4.1 The pituitary–gonadal axis interrupted by castration. 5% of residual androgens are derived from the adrenals.

Once within the prostate, both testosterone and the adrenal androgens are rapidly metabolized by 5-alpha reductase (5-alpha R; an enzyme which is located mainly on the nuclear membrane), to dihydrotestosterone (DHT). The 5-alpha reduced hormone, DHT, is three to five times more potent as an androgen than testosterone itself. Its androgenic action is accomplished in the nucleus by a physical association with androgen receptors which are located mainly on the nuclear membrane. The binding of DHT to the androgen receptor liberates heat-shock protein (hsp90), and unmasks the DNA-binding domain of the receptor, allowing it to dimerize and bind to the specific regulatory sequences, the so-called 'hormone response element' (HRE) of the target genes on the genome. This binding occurs upstream of the transcription start sites of the various androgen-sensitive genes, and thereby stimulates DNA transcription. The messenger RNA molecules (mRNA) thus produced encode a number of proteins, including several important growth factors, such as epidermal growth factor (EGF) and platelet-derived growth factor (PDGF) which modulate prostatic cell growth (**4.2**).

Normal prostate development and maintenance is dependent upon a delicate homeostasis between cell death and cell replacement. Androgens are necessary for this homeostasis, since either medical or surgical castration results in rapid onset of epithelial 'apoptosis' or 'programmed cell death', as well as stromal depletion. The DNA content of androgen-deprived prostatic cells is reduced to 10% within 10 days[2]. Stem cells survive, however, as subsequent replacement of circulating androgens appears capable of restoring both prostatic architecture and function to normal by rapidly switching on the processes concerned with cell proliferation[3].

MOLECULAR CONTROL OF THE CELL CYCLE

Normal prostatic growth and development depends upon a particular pattern of cell division, with some cell types dividing much more often than others, and all divisions occurring in a timely and appropriate fashion.

Prostate epithelial cells divide regularly to maintain the structural integrity of the glandular and ductal epithelial surfaces. The most active epithelial division occurs at the distal tips of the prostate glands; those in the intermediate portion are maintained in a differentiated state undergoing active secretion, and those in the proximal ducts nearest to the urethra undergo programmed cell death (**4.3**).

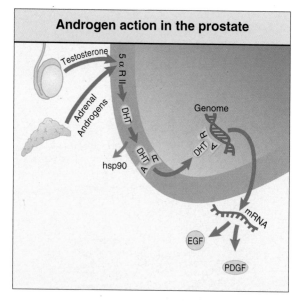

4.2 Androgen activation of androgen-response elements on the genome stimulates transcription and the production of growth factors.

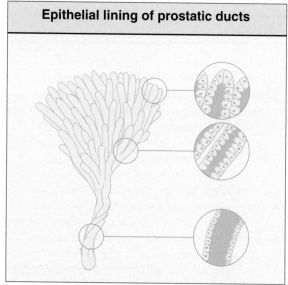

4.3 The arborized prostatic duct system. Cells are produced in the apices of the glands, and migrate down the ductal system undergoing programmed cell death (apoptosis) in the proximal ducts nearest the urethra.

This active process of apoptosis which balances new cell formation is also seen after androgen deprivation; it is currently the subject of much research. The principal morphological feature of apoptosis is the condensation of chromatin caused by production of 180–200 base pair DNA fragments, resulting from the activation of endonucleases[4]. Phosphatase inhibitors appear to synergize with tumour necrosis factor (TNF) to activate DNA fragmentation[5] in this in-built 'cell suicide' system.

CELL DIVISION

The cell-division cycle is traditionally divided into four phases: G1, S, G2 and M (**4.4**). Most differentiated prostatic cells are in G1, which stands for 'gap 1' – when no activity is visible. The S phase denotes the 'synthesis' of DNA, with the cell's chromosomal DNA replicating itself during this phase; this replication process is extremely accurate in that the sequence of the new strands is exactly complementary to the template, and in that every portion of the chromosomal DNA is copied exactly once – no more and no less. The expression of certain genes whose products are needed for DNA replication, such as the histone proteins, is limited exclusively to S phase.

G2 stands for 'gap 2', the second break in visible intracellular activity. At the boundary of S and G2, the replication machinery somehow signals that DNA synthesis is complete; the nature of this signal is unknown, but the cell then enters G2 and prepares itself for mitosis.

The M phase is 'mitosis' – chromosomes condense and become visible as discrete bodies. The two microtubule organizers (or spindle-pole bodies), move apart to opposite sides of the nucleus, and arrays of microtubules grow from the two spindle-pole bodies to form the mitotic spindle. Some of these microtubules become attached to so-called 'kinetochores' on the chromosomes, with the attached chromosomes becoming aligned on the 'metaphase plate' (the plane that lies halfway between the spindle-pole bodies). When all of the kinetochores are attached to microtubules and aligned on the metaphase plate, a biochemical signal is sent, and anaphase begins. The chromosomes start moving towards the poles, and the poles move apart from each other. Finally, the cell pinches in two (cytokinesis), producing two G1-phase daughter cells (**4.5**).

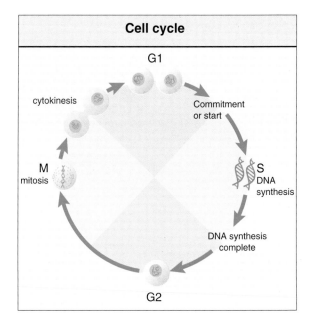

4.4 The cell cycle.

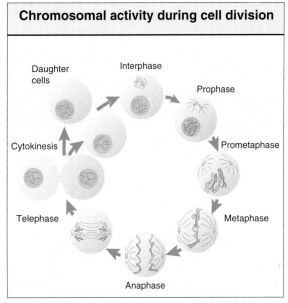

4.5 Chromosomal behaviour during mitosis.

Controls on Cell Division

Controls on the growth of cells within the prostate fall into two categories. First, there are those controls whose regulatory mechanisms influence cell metabolism and enlargement; the normal prostate smooth-muscle cell should neither enlarge nor divide, and should make only enough protein to replace what is lost. The second form of controls influence cell division itself. Epithelial cells within the prostate have a fairly high turnover, but are normally under strict regulation that coordinates both enlargement and cell division.

The nature of both of these controls is currently being elucidated. Molecular biologists have identified and cloned several genes, known collectively as the *Cdc*2 family, whose normal function is necessary for cell division to proceed. *Cdc*2 genes appear to encode proteins which are members of the protein kinase family. (A protein kinase is an enzyme that can transfer a phosphate group from adenosine triphosphate (ATP) onto another protein; phosphorylation either increases or decreases the activity of the protein in question, and is a widely used method of regulating protein activity in biological systems[6].) Another protein that is also intimately involved in the control of the cell cycle has been named 'cyclin'[7]; the gene encoding it has also been cloned[8]. This polypeptide appears to form a stable complex with Cdc2 protein, with the binding of cyclin appearing to activate the protein such that Cdc2 has protein-kinase activity only when cyclin is present. The removal of cyclin from the Cdc2 molecule by intracellular proteases inactivates Cdc2 and may be the key event in completing mitosis (**4.6**).

THE INVOLVEMENT OF GROWTH FACTORS

A number of polypeptides [including epidermal growth factor (EGF), basic fibroblast growth factor (bFGF) and platelet-derived growth factor (PDGF) – see **Table 4.1**] have been identified as potent stimulators of prostate growth.

The receptors for these polypeptides reside on the surfaces of both epithelial and stromal cells, and all seem to possess a large extracellular ligand-binding domain, a single membrane-spanning helix, and a sizable cytoplasmic domain. The cytoplasmic domain is usually an enzyme in the form of a ligand-stimulated protein kinase; these important enzymes are capable of transferring phosphate to tyrosine residues of other proteins. EGF receptors are linked to protein-kinase enzymes and appear to work in pairs or so-called 'dimers', which are produced by EGF binding that induces the receptors to pair off ('dimerize') and to phosphorylate each other. This, in turn, appears to result in the recruitment of several cellular enzymes to the cytoplasmic domain of the receptor. These recruits include enzymes that are involved in the production of phospholipid second messengers, and perhaps of

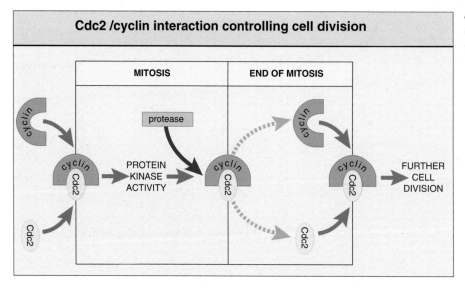

Cdc2 /cyclin interaction controlling cell division

MITOSIS | END OF MITOSIS

cyclin
protease
cyclin
Cdc2
PROTEIN KINASE ACTIVITY
cyclin
Cdc2
cyclin
Cdc2
FURTHER CELL DIVISION
Cdc2
Cdc2

4.6 The control of cell division by Cdc2 and cyclin interaction.

other protein kinases, thus amplifying and distributing the signal within the cell. By these means, the genes controlling growth (such as the *Cdc2* and cyclin families) are turned on, various key proteins are synthetized, and prostatic cell division occurs (**4.7**).

PUTATIVE EVENTS LEADING TO PROSTATE CANCER

Invasive prostate cancer develops when a mutation (or a series of mutations) occurs within a single cell, and gives it a growth advantage over its neighbours. As the number of descendants of the original mutant increases, so does the likehood that one of these will sustain a further mutation that in turn allows its descendants to grow even faster. This deadly cycle of dedifferentiation continues as cells accumulate additional mutations that allow them to accelerate their growth further and to start invading surrounding tissues. Further mutations then permit metastasis – the dangerous propensity of certain prostate cancers to escape and seed new tumours elsewhere in the body, especially in bone. Although the individual events on the road to prostate cancer are rare, men in developed countries now have an increasingly long lifespan and chance dictates that from time to time this lethal stepwise combination of events will unfold.

ACTIVATION OF ONCOGENES

The discovery that DNA tumour viruses are capable of transforming cells by inserting their own genes (which are capable of inducing cell growth and division) into the host genome, and the knowledge that this genetic material is stably transferred to daughter cells, led to the search for so-called 'viral oncogenes'. It subsequently became apparent that inactive forms of similar genes – proto-oncogenes – were in fact present in almost all mammalian cells. These proto-oncogenes encode the proteins involved with various forms of intercellular and intracellular signal transduction, including those of growth factors. But how do these proto-oncogenes become activated to produce virulent oncogenes? The answer to this question came from the study of the *c-ras* gene in bladder cancer, rather than prostate cancer. Comparison of the normal, cloned *c-ras* gene and the activated oncogene revealed only the subtlest of differences: a guanidine nucleotide had been substituted by a thymidine in the oncogene. This mutation changed the twelfth codon of the *ras* gene from a codon encoding glycine to one encoding another amino acid, valine (**4.8**). It became clear that it was this single base-pair change that was the driving force that induced these cells to form bladder tumours.

Table 4.1 Growth factors identified in the prostate
Epidermal growth factor (EGF)
Insulin-like growth factors I and II (IGF I, II)
Keratinocyte growth factor (KGF)
Transforming growth factor alpha (TGF α)
Transforming growth factor beta (TGF β)
Basic fibroblast growth factor (bFGF)

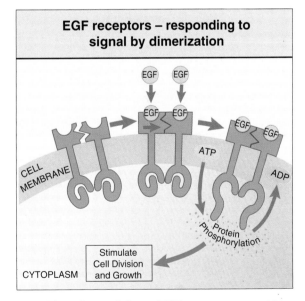

4.7 Epidermal growth factor (EGF) receptors respond to EGF signal by dimerization and autophosphorylation. This process results in the production of phospholipid second messengers which amplify the signal within the cell.

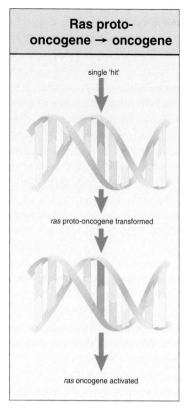

Ras proto-oncogene → oncogene

single 'hit'

ras proto-oncogene transformed

ras oncogene activated

4.8 A single base-pair alteration in the *ras* oncogene bestows carcinogenic properties.

The Mechanisms of Action of Oncogenes

Oncogenes have diverse mechanisms of action. The *ras* gene is part of a larger family of genes encoding guanidine nucleotide-binding proteins, the so-called 'G proteins'. The G proteins are molecular switches that regulate a number of signal transduction pathways, including the alpha-1 adrenoceptor smooth-muscle response within the prostate. They are in their active conformation when bound to a molecule of high-energy guanosine trinucleotide (GTP), and possess an intrinsic enzyme activity that hydrolyses bound GTP to its lower-energy form, guanosine dinucleotide (GDP), returning the G proteins to their ground state. The mutation in the activated *ras* oncogene (**4.8**) destroys this GTP hydrolysis activity, thereby locking the protein in its active conformation (**4.9**).

Other proto-oncogenes act as growth factors. For example, the *sis* oncogene encodes a form of PDGF, the potent mitogen for mesechymal cells to which prostate cells respond. In tissue culture, cells infected with a *sis*-carrying virus become transformed via autocrine stimulation. That is, they secrete a growth factor to which they can also respond. Thus, the cells bathe themselves continually in a factor that makes them grow and divide. Other oncogenes encode altered receptors that trigger growth signals even in

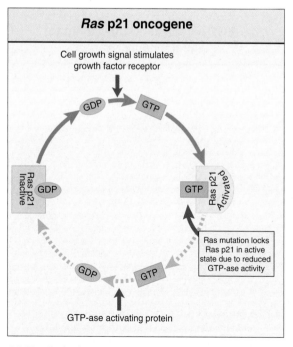

Ras p21 oncogene

Cell growth signal stimulates growth factor receptor

GDP

GTP

Ras p21 Inactive — GDP

GTP — Ras p21 Activated

Ras mutation locks Ras p21 in active state due to reduced GTP-ase activity

GDP — GTP

GTP-ase activating protein

4.9 The 'locked on' *ras* p21 oncogene continually stimulates cell proliferation.

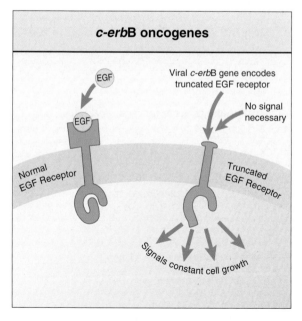

*c-erb*B oncogenes

EGF

EGF

Normal EGF Receptor

Viral *c-erb*B gene encodes truncated EGF receptor

No signal necessary

Truncated EGF Receptor

Signals constant cell growth

4.10 The *erb*B oncogene, when mutated, has a truncated cell-surface receptor. This abnormal receptor continually stimulates cell growth without the requirement of an EGF signal being present.

the absence of ligand. The viral c-erbB gene, for example, encodes a truncated form of EGF receptor that is reduced at each end. In particular, its entire extracellular binding domain has been lopped off. This decapitated receptor acts as if it is constantly responding to ligand EGF, and therefore sends constant growth promoting signals to the interior of the cell in spite of an absence of signal (4.10). A subset of human prostate cancers has been shown to express the c-erbB oncogene in immunohistochemical assays[9].

The largest class of oncogenes is still the least well understood. These encode proteins that occupy the location just inside the plasma membrane. As mentioned previously, protein-tyrosine kinases are intimately involved in the control mechanisms of cell division. The very large number of oncogenic protein-tyrosine kinases confirms that tyrosine phosphorylation is a critical event in growth control. Their individual functions are currently being elucidated.

The proto-oncogenes c-myc, c-fos and c-jun all encode proteins concerned with the regulation of gene transcription[10]. They represent some of the earliest genes to be expressed in the prostate of castrated rats after administration of androgens[11]. These proto-oncogenes transduce the extranuclear mitogenic signals into the expression of genes that then encode the transcription factors – the fos, jun, and myc proteins, which regulate the secondary genes concerned with growth. The fos and jun proteins bind to activating protein (AP-1), which is intimately involved in the regulatory processes controlling cell growth and differentiation. EGF and FGF both induce c-fos and c-jun genes, which have stimulatory effects unless the inhibitory influence of factors such as TGF-beta prevails. In this finely tuned and complex regulatory process, the fos and jun proteins autoregulate the expression of their own genes.

A very large number of oncogenes have now been identified and cloned, and some have been implicated in prostatic cancer[12,13]. In virtually every case, oncogene proteins lie on the signalling pathways by which cells receive and execute cell growth and division instructions. The mutations that activate these genes are either structural mutations that lead to the stimulatory activity of a protein without an incoming signal, or regulatory mutations that lead to the production of the protein at the wrong place or time. Damage to oncogenes thus gives the cell a persistent internal growth signal – the so-called 'autocrine signal' – in the absence of any external stimuli.

Tumour-Suppressor Genes (Anti-Oncogenes)

As oncogene research has progressed, it has become apparent that there exist naturally genes that have the ability to overpower oncogenes and thereby keep them in check. These have been termed anti-oncogenes, or 'tumour-suppressor genes', with the best example being the retinoblastoma (RB) gene. Inherited or acquired mutation of this gene, which is located on chromosome 13, results in the development of retinal tumours in childhood. The RB protein, encoded by the RB gene, has the capability of keeping cell growth in check; certain oncogene viruses act by negating the effect of this protein, thus removing the 'brakes' on cell growth. A mutant protein, expressed as a result of an exon deletion of the RB gene, has been reported in the DU145 prostatic cancer cell line[14]. Moreover, transfection of the cloned, normal RB gene into the tumour cells in nude mice suppressed tumorigenicity. There is evidence that the RB protein may regulate c-myc expression such that levels of myc protein are controlled. Loss of the RB gene and its supressor protein would consequently lead to myc activation and enhanced cell proliferation. Allelic deletions on chromosome 13, the location of the RB gene, have been reported in some patients with prostate cancer[15,16].

Another important example of a tumour-suppressor gene is the p53 gene, the absence of which leads to a dramatically increased incidence of various forms of cancer[17] (4.11). The relatively small size of the p53 gene when compared to the RB gene means that it is a gene with which molecular biologists can work more easily. Various reports have described p53 alterations in prostate-cancer tissue, with most studies suggesting an incidence in 6–20% of specimens tested[18,19]. However, there are several reports describing alterations in up to 80% of specimens analysed[20]. It appears that p53 mutations tend to appear more often in late-stage hormone-resistant tumours. This event may therefore be involved in the final stages of prostatic oncogenesis.

THE STEP-WISE DEVELOPMENT OF PROSTATE CANCER

The epidemiology of many human tumours has long suggested that cancer is a multistep process in which the genome is sequentially subjected to a number of random 'hits'. Statistical calculations based upon the increasing frequency of cancer with age have estimated the number of these steps or 'hits' to be between four and six. As already discussed, about 9% of prostate cancers appear to be the result of an inherited tendency[21]. Inheritance of this disease leads to a greater than two-fold increase in the risk of developing prostate cancer, and those tumours that do develop do so at an unusually young age. Chromosomal mapping of

affected families is currently underway, and cytogenetic studies have shown chromosomal abnormalities in association with prostate cancer at 7q, 8p, 10q, 16q, and 18q loci.

The oncogene *her*-2 has also been found to be associated with prostate cancer[9]. Elevated *c-myc* mRNA levels have also been demonstrated in prostate cancer,

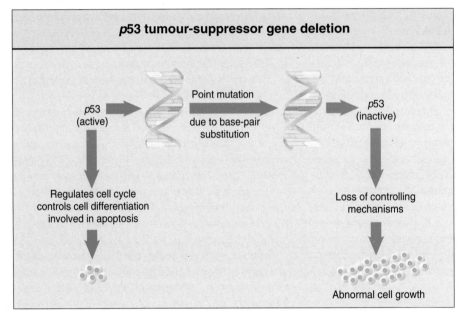

4.11 Mutation of the *p53* tumour-suppressor gene results in loss of controlling mechanisms and promotes abnormal cell growth.

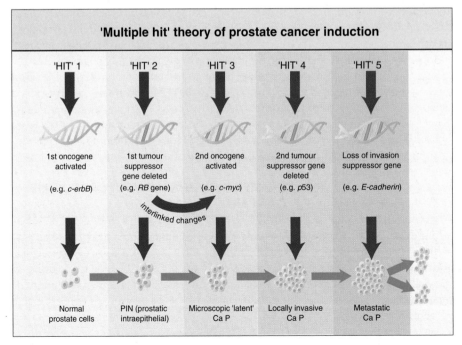

4.12 A schematic representation of the 'multiple hit' theory of the induction of prostate cancer.

with suggestions that higher concentrations relate to higher-grade cancer. A proposed order of events in the development of prostate cancer is illustrated in **4.12**. These are certainly not the sole or specific events involved, and the order of their occurence is not critical. It is the accumulation of events resulting in what has been described as 'a complementary misbehaviour of genes', rather than their order, that counts in terms of tumour development[22].

MOLECULAR FACTORS INFLUENCING THE DEVELOPMENT OF METASTASES

For a prostate cancer cell to metastasize (usually to bone or, less commonly, soft tissue), it has to acquire the ability to migrate from its original site and to grow and divide in a new environment. The molecular events involved in producing this lethal tendency are currently under intense scutiny[23]. One factor may be the loss of cell-adhesion molecules such as E-cadherin, which normally binds cells together. The gene for E-cadherin, which has been termed an 'invasion suppressor gene', is located on chromosome 16q. In human cancer specimens, a correlation was found between E-cadherin expession and the Gleason grade of the tumour[24]. A correlation of E-cadherin expression and survival of patients with prostate cancer is also apparent.

Other features relating to the metastatic potential of a given prostatic tumour include the ability of cells to invade tissues by local secretion of collagenase enzymes. In addition, as mentioned in Chapter 2, prostate cancer metastases require a local blood supply to sustain themselves[25] (**4.13**). The release of peptides that stimulate the growth of new blood vessels (angiogenesis factors) may be important in this respect, and these themselves possibly act in synergy with local growth factors such as bFGF[26,27]. Recent studies also suggest the presence of an antimetastatic nm23 protein, encoded by the *nm23* gene, located on chromosome 17[28,29]. Loss of this restraining influence may be one of several further factors in determining the presence of the lethal tendency of a given tumour to spread.

FACTORS INFLUENCING THE DEVELOPMENT OF ANDROGEN INDEPENDENCE

Androgen-dependent cells undergo apoptosis and die in the absence of hormone, whereas androgen-sensitive cells can survive in the absence of androgen stimulus, but grow more quickly in its presence. In addition, some cells may be indirectly dependent upon androgens, requiring paracrine growth-promoting factors from neighbouring androgen-sensitive cells. It is presumed that the automatous growth of androgen-independent cells occurs by clonal selection and results in cancer progression. But it is not inconceivable that androgen-sensitive cells adapt to lower levels of androgen by means of the constitutive expression of growth-related oncogenes, a factor we shall consider later in relation to the use of maximum androgen blockade versus monotherapy (see Chapter 13). Genetic instability of a developing tumour could easily lead to the formation of cell variants with different degrees of sensitivity to androgen, including the production of androgen receptor mutants akin to the situation with oestrogen receptors in breast cancer[30]. Androgen receptor mutants are well recognized as a cause of congenital androgen-insensitivity syndrome, and a mutant receptor has been identified in one variant of the LNCaP prostate-cancer cell line[31]. In this case, the changes in ligand specificity were such that growth responses could be elicited by the administration of antiandrogens.

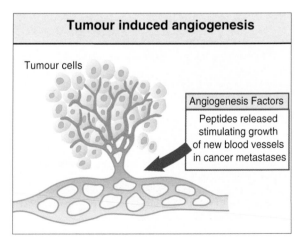

Tumour induced angiogenesis

Tumour cells

Angiogenesis Factors

Peptides released stimulating growth of new blood vessels in cancer metastases

4.13 The ability of tumour cells to metastasize is dependent upon their capacity to induce their own blood supply; this process is known as angiogenesis, and may develop in response to secreted angiogenesis factors.

TO WHAT EXTENT DOES MOLECULAR BIOLOGICAL KNOWLEDGE TRANSLATE INTO IMPROVED PATIENT CARE?

Although the recent exponential increase in our understanding of the molecular biology of cancer has yet to translate into improved patient care, the seeds of change are already present and are now growing fast. As our knowledge improves, the possibility of preventing prostate cancer by the use of agents such as retinoids or 5-alpha reductase inhibitors that block some of the molecular events on the road to cancer seems feasible. Early detection, already possible by means of prostate specific antigen (PSA) assay, may certainly be enhanced by the development of newer, more cancer-specific, tumour markers. In addition, chromosomal mapping is likely to identify the genes responsible for familial prostate cancer, and to provide a means of confirming a need for increased cancer surveillance in certain individuals. Improved staging, utilizing polymerase chain technology (PCR) to amplify tiny amounts of metastatic tumour DNA or mRNA, may help to identify those patients whose disease is already beyond hope of purely local therapies. 'Gene therapy' for prostate cancer is still some way off, but the possibilities of replacing tumour-suppressor genes, neutralizing oncogenes, and specifically enhancing the immune responses to a given prostate cancer now appear attainable (see Chapter 14). The limitations of androgen-deprivation therapy may be circumvented by the development of more specific growth factor, metastatic or angiogenesis inhibitors[32]. Many of these latest developments and future possibilities in these exciting areas are discussed in subsequent chapters.

REFERENCES

1 Crawford ED, Eisenberger MA, McLeod DG, et al. A controlled trial of leuprolide with and without flutamide in prostatic cancer. N Engl J Med 1989;**321**:419–424.

2 Bruchovsky N, Lesser B, Van Doorn E, et al. Hormonal effects on cell proliferation in rat prostate. Vitam Horm 1975;**33**:61–102.

3 Isaacs JT. Antagonistic effect of androgen on prostatic cell death. Prostate 1984;**5**:545–557.

4 Oberhammer F, Wilson JW, Dive C, et al. Apoptotic death in epithelial cells: cleavage of DNA to 300 and/or 50 kb fragments prior to or in the absence of internucleosomal fragmentation. The EMBO Journal 1993;**12 (9)**:3679–3684.

5 Wright SC, Zheng H, Zhong J, et al. Role of protein phosphorylation in TNF-induced apoptosis: phosphatase inhibitors synergize with TNF to activate DNA fragmentation in normal as well as TNF-resistant U937 variants. J Cell Biochem 1993;**53**:222–223.

6 Nurse P. Universal control mechanism controlling onset of M phase. Nature 1990;**344**:503–508.

7 Evans TE, Rosenthal J, Youngblom D, et al. Cyclin: a protein specified by maternal mRNA in sea urchin eggs that is destroyed at each cleavage division. Cell 1993;**33**:389–396.

8 Motokura T, Bloom T, Kim HG, et al. A novel cyclin encoded by a bcl1-linked candidate oncogene. Nature 1991;**350**:512–515.

9 Zhau HE, Wan DS, Zhou J, et al. Expression of c-erbB-2/neu proto-oncogene in human prostatic cancer tissues and cell lines. Mol Carc 1992;**5**:320–327.

10 Evan GL, Littlewood TD. The role of c-myc in cell growth [Review]. Current Opinion in Genetics & Development 1993;**3(1)**:44–49.

11 Katz AE, Benson MC, Wise GJ, et al. Gene activity during the early phase of androgen-stimulated rat prostate regrowth. Canc Res 1989;**49(21)**:5889–5894.

12 Schalken JA, Bussemakers MJG, Debruyne FMJ. Oncogene expression in prostate cancer. Oncogenes 1990;**7**:97–105.

13 Klotz LH, Auger M, Andrulis I, et al. Molecular analysis of neu, sis, c-myc, fos, and P53 oncogenes in benign prostatic hypertrophy and prostatic carcinoma. J Urol 1990;**143**:401A.

14 Bookstein R, Rio P, Madreperla SA, et al. Promoter deletion and loss of retinoblastoma gene expression in human prostate carcinoma. Proc Natl Acad Sci 1990;**87**:7762–7766.

15 Brooks JD, Bova GS, Marshall FF, et al. Allelic losses of retinoblastoma gene in primary renal and prostate cancers. J Urol 1993;**149**:376A(652).

16 Sarkar FH, Sakr W, Li YW, et al. Analysis of retinoblastoma (RB) gene deletion in human prostatic carcinoma. Prostate 1992;**21**:145–152.

17 Hollstein M, Sidransky D, Vogelstein B, et al. p53 mutations in human cancers. Science 1991;**253**:49–53.

18 Van Veldhuizen PJ, Sadasivan R, Garcia F, et al. Mutant p53 expression in prostate carcinoma. Prostate 1993;**22**:23–30.

19 Bookstein R, MacGrogan D, Sharkey F, et al. p53 mutations in human prostate cancer. Proc Am Assoc Cancer Res 1993;**34**:537–543.

20 de Vere White RW, Gumerlock PH, Chi SG, et al. p53 tumour suppression gene abnormalities are frequent in human prostate tissues. J Urol 1993;**149**:376A–(654).

21 Isaacs WB, Carter BS. Genetic changes associated with prostate cancer in humans. Cancer Surveys 1991;**11**:15–23.

22 Weinberg RA. Oncogenes, antioncogenes, and the molecular basis of multistep carcinogenesis. Canc Res 1989;**49**:3713–3732.

23 Steeg PS, Bevaliaqua G, Kopper L, et al. Evidence for a novel gene associated with low tumor metastatic potential. J Natl Cancer Inst 1988;**80(3)**:200–204.

24 Umbas R, Schalken JA, Aalders TW, et al. Expression of cellular adhesion molecule E-cadherin is reduced or absent in high-grade prostate cancer. Canc Res 1992;**52**:5104–5109.

25 Myers C, Trepel J, Sartor O, et al. Predictors of pathologic stage in prostatic carcinoma. The role of neovascularity. Cancer 1993;**71 (3)**:1172–1178.

26 Wakui S, Furusato M, Itoh T, *et al.* Tumour angiogenesis in prostatic carcinoma with and without bone marrow metastasis: a morphometric study. *J Pathol* 1992;**168**:257–262.

27 Weidner N, Carroll PR, Flax J, *et al.* Tumour angiogenesis correlates with metastasis in invasive prostate carcinoma. *Am J Pathol* 1993;**143**:401–409.

28 Leone A, Flatow U, Vanlloutte K, *et al.* Transfection of human nm23-H1 into the human MDA-MB-435 breast carcinoma cell line: effects on tumor metastatic potential, colonization and enzymatic activity. *Oncogene* 1993;**8(9)**:2325–2333.

29 Stahl JA, Leone A, Rosengard AM, *et al.* Identification of a second human nm23 gene, nm23-H2. *Canc Res* 1991;**51(1)**:445–449.

30 King RJ. Progression from steroid sensitive to insensitive state in breast tumours. *Cancer Surveys* 1992;**14**:131–146.

31 French FS, Lubahn DB, Brown TR, *et al.* Molecular basis of androgen insensitivity [Review]. *Recent Progress in Hormone Research* 1990;**46**:1–38; discussion 38–42.

32 Yamoaka M, Yamamoto T, Ikeyama S, *et al.* Angiogenesis inhibitor TNP-470 (AGM-1470) potentially inhibits the tumour growth of hormone-independent human breast and prostate carcinoma cell lines. *Canc Res* 1993;**53**:5233–5236.

CHAPTER 5

CLINICAL DIAGNOSIS

INTRODUCTION

The pattern of presentation of prostate cancer changed little until a decade ago; since then there has been a pronounced 'downward' stage migration towards earlier stage disease. This change has been driven by increasing knowledge of the condition, awareness of the dangers of neglecting symptoms, and increasing attempts to detect the condition early, especially using the serum marker, prostate specific antigen (PSA). In the first three quarters of this century, a large proportion of men with clinically significant prostate cancer presented with the symptom complex of weight loss, bone pain, lethargy (due to anaemia and uraemia) and bladder outflow symptoms, all attributable to either locally advanced or metastatic prostate cancer. Pros-

tate cancer still does present in this way in many men beyond middle-age, but now it is increasingly being detected at an earlier stage (**5.1**). This earlier presentation not infrequently confronts both the urologist and primary-care physician with a dilemma concerning treatment, since it is not always clear (especially in the elderly) whether the tumour will progress within the natural lifespan of the individual in which it is found.

PRESENTING SYMPTOMS

Men with prostate cancer can present with a variety of different symptoms, and often with no symptoms at all. Screening for prostate cancer in the asymptomatic male is such a complex and controversial issue that

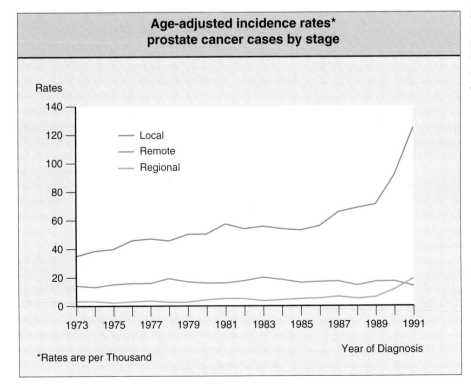

5.1 Age-adjusted incidence rates of prostate cancer in Detroit by stage. Note the recent rapid increase in localized cancers. (SEER data.)

an entire chapter of this book is devoted to this subject (see Chapter 6). However, few would deny that an inquisitive, asymptomatic patient over the age of 45, with concerns about prostate cancer, should receive some basic investigations, if only to reassure him that there is little chance that he does in fact have prostate cancer. The investigation of asymptomatic men with a family history of prostate cancer in one or more first degree relatives seems likely soon to become standard practice.

The presenting symptoms of men with prostate cancer can be broadly divided into:

- Bladder outflow obstruction symptoms.
- Symptoms attributable to local extension of the tumour (e.g. haematuria, ureteric obstruction causing loin pain, etc.).
- Symptoms from metastases (e.g. bone pain and weight loss).

The most frequently encountered presenting symptoms are outlined in **Table 5.1** and **5.3**.

Symptoms of Bladder Outflow Obstruction

The majority of men with prostate cancer will have concomitant histological, benign prostatic hyperplasia (BPH). Although in some cases outflow-obstruction symptoms may be attributable to the cancer (especially if it is locally advanced), in many cases the BPH, which arises within the transition zone close to the prostatic urethra, is much more likely to cause

Table 5.1 Presenting symptoms of localized prostate cancer	
Local	Poor stream Hesitancy Sensation of incomplete emptying Frequency Urgency Urge incontinence
Locally invasive	Haematuria Dysuria Pain Impotence Incontinence Loin pain (ureteric obstruction) Symptoms of renal failure Rectal symptoms including bleeding Haemospermia

lower urinary tract symptoms. Since prostate cancer most often arises in the peripheral zone, it is less likely to cause obstructive symptoms until it is of considerable volume, and by which time will also be extra-capsular. It is interesting to note that in spite of exhaustive pre-operative investigation, approximately 10% of men undergoing transurethral resection (TURP) for supposed BPH are found to have foci of prostate cancer within the resected chips. It is unlikely that such small volume 'sub-clinical' prostate cancers contribute significantly to outflow obstruction.

Bladder outflow obstruction symptoms have been extensively investigated in BPH, and symptom scores devised by the American Urologic Association[1] endorsed by the World Health Organization; these are shown in **Table 5.2**. Although primarily designed to evaluate patients with BPH and their response to various treatments, the International Prostate Symptom Score (IPSS) (**Table 5.2**) can also be used to measure the severity of obstructive and irritative lower urinary tract symptoms in prostate cancer, and also to gauge response to local and systemic treatments.

The symptoms of bladder outflow obstruction are usefully divided into two groups: obstructive and irritative. Obstructive symptoms, namely reduced uroflow, hesitancy and incomplete emptying, result from occlusion of the prostatic urethra by tumour. Urinary retention – the ultimate obstructive symptom – is a common occurrence in locally advanced prostate cancer; it necessitates urgent decompression by either urethral or suprapubic catheterization. Irritative symptoms such as urinary frequency and urgency result from secondary detrusor instability as a response to obstruction and are usually due to BPH; they may, however, also occur with prostate cancer. In addition, irritative symptoms may occur in prostate cancer because of invasion of the trigone of the bladder and pelvic nerves.

Bladder outflow obstruction may lead to secondary problems such as recurrent urinary tract infections, which in turn result in frequency, dysuria and sometimes also haematuria. Urinary stasis within the bladder can result in the formation of bladder calculi, which can themselves predispose the patient to recurrent urinary sepsis (**5.2**). Irritation of the trigone by stones may cause suprapubic pain, strangury and haematuria, especially towards the end of micturition. Haemospermia is a symptom that is only occasionally associated with prostate cancer, but the description of this by a patient should prompt both a digital rectal examination with PSA determination and transrectal ultrasonography.

Table 5.2 International Prostate Symptom Score (IPSS)

Patient Name: Date:	Not at all	Less than 1 time in 5	Less than half the time	About half the time	More than half the time	Almost always
1. Incomplete emptying Over the past month, how often have you had a sensation of not emptying your bladder completely after you finish urinating?	0	1	2	3	4	5
2. Frequency Over the past month, how often have you had to urinate again less than two hours after you finished urinating?	0	1	2	3	4	5
3. Intermittency Over the past month, how often have you found you stopped and started again several times when you urinated?	0	1	2	3	4	5
4. Urgency Over the past month, how often have you found it difficult to postpone urination?	0	1	2	3	4	5
5. Weak stream Over the past month, how often have you had a weak urinary stream?	0	1	2	3	4	5
6. Straining Over the past month, how often have you had to push or strain to begin urination?	0	1	2	3	4	5

	None	1 time	2 times	3 times	4 times	5 times or more
7. Nocturia Over the past month, how many times did you most typically get up to urinate from the time you went to bed at night until the time you got up in the morning?	0	1	2	3	4	5

	Delighted	Pleased	Mostly Satisfied	Mixed-about equally satisfied and dissatisfied	Mostly Dissatisfied	Unhappy	Terrible
Quality of life due to urinary symptoms If you were to spend the rest of your life with your urinary condition just the way it is now, how would you feel about that?	0	1	2	3	4	5	6

The International Prostate Symptom Score (IPSS) is based on the answers to seven questions concerning urinary symptoms. Each question is assigned points from 0 to 5 indicating increasing severity of the particular symptom. The total score can range from 0 to 35 (asymptomatic to very symptomatic). Although there are presently no standard recommendations for grading patients with mild, moderate or severe symptoms, patients can be tentatively classified as follows: **0–7 = mildly symptomatic; 8–19 = moderately symptomatic; 20–35 = severely symptomatic.** The International Consensus Committee (ICC) recommends the use of only a single question to assess a patient's quality of life. The answers to this question range from 'delighted' to 'terrible', or 0–6. Although this single question may or may not capture the global impact of BPH symptoms on quality of life, it can serve as a valuable starting point for a doctor–patient conversation.

Symptoms of Local Invasion

Carcinomatous infiltration within the prostate and local invasion of adjacent structures can lead to an assortment of symptoms. Direct invasion of the prostatic urethra may lead to haematuria, which may on occasions be profuse with clots. The haematuria may be associated with dysuria due to malignant infiltration of the urothelium within the prostatic urethra.

Urinary incontinence may be a consequence of local invasion of the distal urethral sphincter mechanism, which may be so debilitating that it necessitates permanent catheterization. It is, however, important to be sure in such circumstances that incontinence is not due to chronic retention with overflow, which could potentially be remedied by TURP or by other local therapeutic procedures such as intraprostatic stent insertion.

Extracapsular posterolateral extension of prostate cancer may lead to invasion and destruction of the neurovascular bundles, and erectile impotence (see 2.5). It is important to bear this unusual presentation of prostate cancer in mind when investigating men of middle-age or beyond for symptoms of erectile dysfunction. Extracapsular extension of cancer may also invade other nerves, leading to pain which is characteristically located in the perineum and suprapubic areas. This differential diagnosis should be borne in mind when investigating prostatitis. Invasion of the seminal vesicles may result in haemospermia.

Extension of prostate cancer posteriorly can lead to lower bowel symptoms and, rarely, prostate cancer may present in such a way. The fascia of Denonvillier is generally protective against direct invasion of the rectal wall by prostate cancer, but it is not unknown for

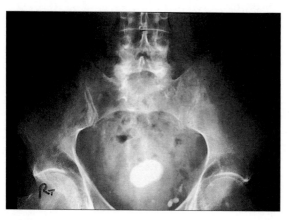

5.2 A bladder stone seen on plain x-ray.

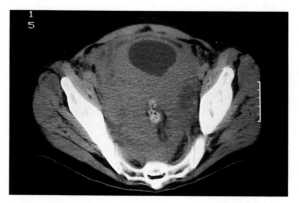

5.3 CT scan showing an enormous prostate cancer encircling the rectum; this patient presented with subacute large bowel obstruction.

Table 5.3 Presenting symptoms of metastatic prostate cancer	
Local metastatic	Bone pain (consider pathological fracture when acute) Paraplegia (secondary to cord compression) Lymph node enlargement Lymphoedema (particularly lower limb) Loin pain (ureteric obstruction)
Systemic metastatic	Lethargy (due to anaemia, uraemia and non-specific effects) Weight loss and cachexia Haemorrhage (cutaneous and bowel)

locally advanced prostate cancer to encircle the distal rectum completely, leading eventually to large bowel obstruction (**5.3**). Prostate cancer patients presenting in this way may be erroneously referred to the colorectal clinic with symptoms such as constipation and rectal bleeding. At sigmoidoscopy, the tumour may mimic a primary rectal tumour and biopsy will show adenocarcinoma. In such circumstances, specific immunohistochemical PSA staining of the biopsies will identify the prostate as the origin of the tumour (**2.27**), and serum PSA will almost always be markedly elevated.

Symptoms of Metastatic Disease

Internationally, in spite of efforts to detect early disease by increasing the public awareness of symptoms attributable to prostate diseases and the screening of asymptomatic men (see Chapter 7), considerably more than 40% of men with prostate cancer still present with spread of disease beyond the confines of the prostate.

Currently, in Europe, at least a quarter of men with prostate cancer will also have bone metastases detectable on an isotope bone scan at presentation[2]. These individuals may have a number of symptoms (**Table 5.3**). Local pain is the commonest symptom caused by bone metastases, and since these are most frequently found within the pelvic bones and lumbar spine, sudden onset of progressive, low-back pain is a cardinal symptom of metastatic prostate cancer. Bony metastases from prostate cancer may be seen in almost every bone in the skeleton, and can lead to pathological fractures, especially as a result of local trauma. The neck of the femur is not an uncommon site for metastatic prostate cancer, and is particularly prone to pathological fracture, often necessitating orthopaedic surgical correction by prosthetic arthroplasty. Acute, severe, hip pain, and inability to bear weight on the affected limb in an elderly male with bladder outflow symptoms, suggests this diagnosis. Metastatic disease within the vertebral bodies is common in prostate cancer, and compression of the spinal cord causing neurological symptoms (especially within the lower limbs) may occur in 1–12% of patients[3] (**5.4**); in one series, in 17% of cases of acute spinal-cord compression due to metastatic prostate cancer, this was the initial presentation of the disease[4]. Although opinions are divided between the comparative benefits of radiotherapy and surgical decompression, it is important to emphasize the importance of prompt treatment in all cases of cord compression that is secondary to bony metastases, in order to achieve a propitious therapeutic outcome[5]. Extensive metastatic disease within the bone marrow may lead to normochromic, normocytic anaemia, due to both the replacement of marrow as well as to cachexia.

While metastatic prostate cancer within the skeleton may present with dramatic symptoms, the presentation of lymph-node metastases is usually less overt. Enlarging nodal masses may become apparent to the patient, particularly within the inguinal lymph nodes, but also occasionally within the cervical and axillary nodes. Intra-abdominal, lymphatic, metastatic spread initially involves the obturator and internal iliac lymph nodes, and may result in ureteric obstruction. Later, tumour may spread to common iliac, external iliac, inguinal and para-aortic nodes; eventually, lymphatic involvement may spread as far as thoracic, cervical and axillary lymph node chains. Lymphatic involvement from prostate cancer may cause a variety of symptoms, including palpable swellings noticed by the patient, loin pain due to upper urinary tract obstruction, and lymphoedematous lower limb swelling.

Spinal metastases–spinal cord compression

5.4 Spinal-cord compression resulting from metastases of prostate cancer in the lumbar spine.

PHYSICAL EXAMINATION

Routine, external physical examination may reveal no abnormality suggesting an underlying diagnosis of prostatic carcinoma. However, since prostate cancer is such a commonly encountered disease in men (and especially in the older male), not only urologists but also primary health-care physicians should be aware of the salient physical signs that should alert their attention towards this important diagnosis. More precise physical examination is usually guided by the presenting medical history, and hence, symptoms of bladder outflow obstruction should raise a suspicion of underlying prostate cancer. On physical examination, the search for prostate cancer should include an inspection for bladder distension (assisted by percussion of the lower abdomen), as well as examination of the lower limbs for lymphoedema and lymph nodes for enlargement and induration.

Digital Rectal Examination

Examination of the prostate digitally per rectum (DRE) is still the most useful clinical method for the diagnosis of prostate cancer, provided the tumour is of sufficient volume to be palpable (**5.5**).

The precise technique for examining the prostate varies from one country to another. In the UK, patients are usually examined in the left lateral position with the knees brought up to the chest. In the USA, DRE is more often performed from behind the patient, with the patient standing and leaning forwards. There is little hard evidence to suggest that the positioning of the patient makes much difference in the diagnostic yield of DRE.

It is fortuitous that the majority (approximately 70%) of prostate cancers arise from within the peripheral zone and hence are more likely to be palpable by DRE. In a recent series of 6630 men, DRE detected 55% of prostate cancers while TRUS detected 82%[6]; this difference reflects the impalpability of small prostate

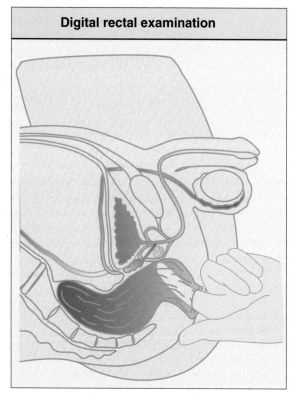

Digital rectal examination

5.5 Digital rectal examination (DRE) of a posteriorly located prostatic nodule.

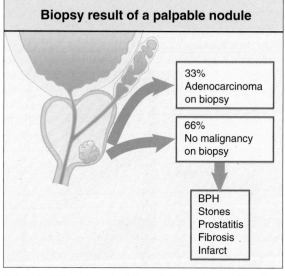

Biopsy result of a palpable nodule

33%
Adenocarcinoma
on biopsy

66%
No malignancy
on biopsy

BPH
Stones
Prostatitis
Fibrosis
Infarct

5.6 Probability of a palpable nodule proving positive for adenocarcinoma on transrectal biopsy.

cancers. However, DRE may suggest a false positive diagnosis of prostate cancer when a firm palpable nodule or induration is felt. Histological examination of such areas reveals prostate cancer in about only one third of cases[7] (**5.6**). The differential diagnoses of such abnormal palpable lesions are summarized in **Table 5.4**.

LOCAL STAGING OF PROSTATE CANCER

Early stages of prostate cancer (T2a or Stage B1), if palpable, appear as a peripheral, firm nodule, that is not apparently distorting the capsule. More extensive cancers (T2b or Stage B2) feel hard and less discrete, with unilateral enlargement when confined to one side of the gland. Stage T3 (Stage C) prostate cancer is again palpably hard; irregular distortion of the prostate outline is often apparent, but the prostate as a whole remains mobile; the seminal vesicles are often involved, and may be palpable. In locally advanced T4 prostate cancer, the prostate is grossly enlarged, hard, irregular throughout, and immobile due to fixation to adjacent structures (**5.7**).

Loss of palpability of the median sulcus of the prostate is a non-specific finding that may be found in T2–T4 disease. BPH can usually be differentiated from prostate cancer on DRE by virtue of the softer, springier, and more symmetrical nature of the benign gland. However, peripheral-zone calcification, which is a common feature of BPH, particularly when associated with chronic prostatitis, may masquerade as prostate cancer since hard and often discrete nodules may be palpable. Acute prostatitis (which may lead to a rise in the PSA and hypoechoic TRUS findings), in which the prostate is soft and exquisitely tender, is easier to differentiate from prostate cancer; chronic prostatitis, particularly granulomatous prostatitis, however, is often clinically indistinguishable[8].

DRE as a Guide to Biopsy

DRE can be used to guide biopsies of the prostate that utilize fine-needle aspiration techniques or trucut/biopty biopsies. It is difficult to guide biopsies of small, palpable lesions digitally, and this technique has largely been superseded by TRUS-guided biopsy with an automatic device. All palpably abnormal lesions should be considered for biopsy, taking into account the patient's age and life expectancy. The decision regarding the necessity for biopsy of the prostate when no suspicious lesions are palpable is guided by the level of serum PSA and the presence or absence of

any abnormal findings on TRUS. This topic is discussed in more detail in the chapters dealing with imaging, PSA and screening. Although misleading in some cases, and not diagnostic for prostate cancer in isolation, DRE remains the crucial first step towards making the diagnosis of prostate cancer. Palpation of the prostate should not be considered as exclusively

Table 5.4 Causes of false positive diagnosis of prostate cancer on digital rectal examination
BPH nodule
Prostatic calculi
Prostatitis
Ejaculatory duct anomaly
Seminal vesicle anomaly
Rectal wall phlebolith
Rectal wall polyp/tumour

Local staging of prostate cancer

T2a (B1)   T2c (B2)

T3c (C1)   T4c (C2)

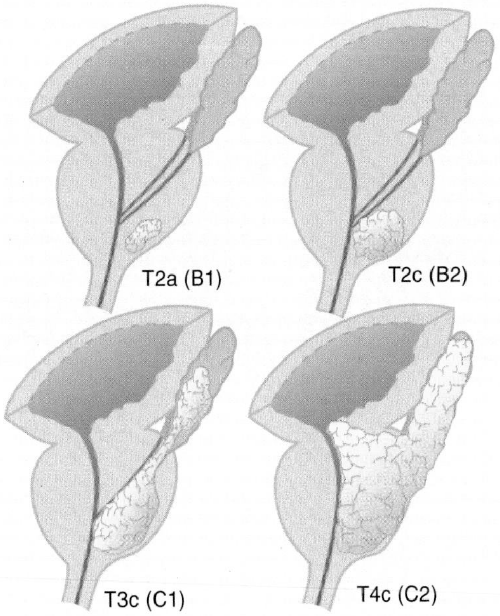

5.7 Local staging of prostate cancer.

within the realm of the urologist. Primary health-care physicians should also be encouraged to develop expertise in DRE, and to use their acquired skill to contribute towards earlier detection of prostate cancer, especially in men under the age of 70 years who are most likely to benefit from this.

Incidental Prostate Cancer

One of the most common presentations of localized prostate cancer remains the 'incidental' diagnosis of the disease at TURP[9]. However, the recent decline in the number of transurethral resections performed for what is presumed to be benign disease, and the increase in the pre-operative PSA testing and ultrasound-guided transrectal prostatic biopsy, seems likely to reduce the frequency with which the larger volume, more clinically significant incidental prostate cancers are diagnosed in this way.

Currently, of those incidental cancers that are detected, roughly two thirds are well-differentiated tumours involving 5% or less of the resected chippings; this has been termed T1a (A1) stage disease. In the remaining one third of cases, there is evidence of less well-differentiated (Gleason grade > 4) tissue and/or involvement of more than 5% of the resected tissue (T1b (A2) stage disease).

Although the T1a/T1b classification is easy to apply clinically, and correlates reasonably well with the subsequent risk of disease progression, it does possess some obvious drawbacks in terms of prognosis for the individual patient. The tissue sampled at TURP is predominantly that of the transition zone, from whence less than 30% of prostate cancers stem. More importantly, the 5% of curettings involved by the 'cancer cut-off point' employed do carry a substantial risk of underestimation, or sometimes overestimation, of the residual disease present after TURP (especially when the disease is multifocal)[10]. The nature of the problem is illustrated in **5.8**.

There may not always be a good correlation between the volume and grade of cancer excised with that of the extent and nature of tumour remaining. However, the means to circumvent this problem are now available: a reasonable estimate of that volume and grade of residual disease can be obtained by postoperative PSA determination and transrectal ultrasound-guided biopsy. Those patients with biopsy-proven residual cancer of a volume > 0.5 cm^3, and who have a life expectancy of more than 10 years, might be considered for definitive therapy – either surgery or radical radiotherapy. By contrast, those with no evidence of significant-volume or high-grade residual

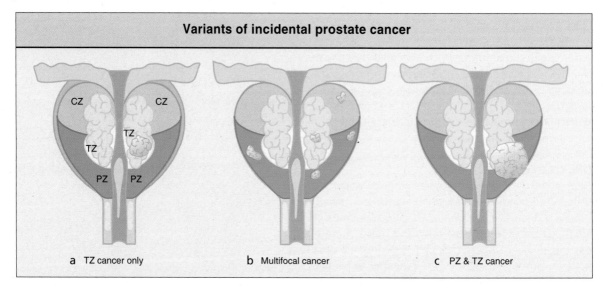

a TZ cancer only   b Multifocal cancer   c PZ & TZ cancer

5.8 Variations in anatomical locations of prostatic tumours diagnosed incidentally at TURP. Case (**a**) the cancer would be completely excised; case (**b**) is multifocal and small residual areas of cancer would remain; case (**c**) TURP simply samples the 'tip of the iceberg' of a larger, predominantly peripheral-zone, cancer.

disease can be managed by so-called 'watchful waiting'[11]. A rise in serum PSA of more than 0.75 ng/ml per annum in men younger than 75 years of age, however, should set alarm bells ringing and should prompt repeat ultrasound-guided transrectal biopsies which, if positive, might suggest the need for further therapy[12].

CONCLUSIONS

Careful history and examination, including, crucially, DRE, remain the cornerstone of the clinical evaluation of patients suspected of harbouring prostate cancer. The diagnosis of prostate cancer, however, may have a profound effect on the affected individual and his family. Caution should therefore be exercised in setting the wheels in motion of confirming the presence of prostate cancer in very elderly men, since active treatment may not always be indicated. In men younger than 75 years whose life expectancy exceeds 5–10 years, however, accurate diagnosis and appropriate therapy may prevent the development of extensive metastatic disease with its severely negative impact on quality of life. A high index of suspicion and diagnosis acumen is necessary to identify correctly those individuals harbouring disease that constitutes a potential threat to their lives at a stage when it is still potentially curable.

REFERENCES

1. Barry MJ, Fowler FJ, O'Leary MP, et al. The American Urologic Association index for benign prostatic hyperplasia. J Urol 1992;**140**:1549–1557.

2. Johansson JE, Adami MD, Andersson SO, et al. Natural history of localised prostate cancer: a population-based study in 223 untreated patients. Lancet 1989;**1**:799–801.

3. Liskow A, Chang CH, De Sanctis P. Epidural cord compression in association with genito-urinary neoplasms. Cancer 1986;**58**:949–954.

4. Rosenthal MA, Rosen D, Raghavan D, et al. Spinal cord compression in prostate cancer. A 10-year experience. Br J Urol 1992;**69**:530–533.

5. Iacovou JW, Marks JC, Abrams P, et al. Cord compression and carcinoma of the prostate; is laminectomy justified? Br J Urol 1985;**57**:733–736.

6. Catalona WJ, Richie JP, Ahmann FR, et al. Comparison of digital rectal examination and serum prostate specific antigen in the early detection of prostate cancer: results of a multicentre clinical trial of 6630 men. J Urol 1994;**151**:1283–1290.

7. Catalona WJ. Yield from routine prostatic needle biopsy in patients more than 50 years old referred for urologic evaluation. J Urol 1980;**124**:844–846.

8. Lui S, Miller PD, Kirby RS. Eosinophilic prostatitis and prostate specific antigen. Br J Urol 1992;**69**:61–63.

9. Matzkin H, Patel JP, Altwein JE, et al. Stage T_{1a} carcinoma of the prostate. Urol 1994;**43**:11–21.

10. Voges GE, McNeal JE, Redwine EA, et al. The predictive significance of substaging stage A prostate cancer (A_1 versus A_2) for volume and grade of total cancer in the prostate. J Urol 1992;**147**:858–863.

11. Cantrell BB, De Klerk DP, Eggleston JC, et al. Pathological factors that influence prognosis in stage A prostatic cancer: the influence of extent versus grade. J Urol 1981;**125**:516–520.

12. Feneley MR, Webb JAW, McLean A, Kirby RS. Post-operative serial prostate-specific antigen and transrectal ultrasound for staging incidental carcinoma of the prostate. Br J Urol 1995;**75**:14–20.

CHAPTER 6

TUMOUR MARKERS IN PROSTATE CANCER

Serum tumour markers are often a most helpful tool in the evaluation and management of patients with any type of neoplasm. While a number of markers have shown clinical utility, a lack of specificity and sensitivity has caused many others that initially generated great interest to fall into disfavour. The increasing application of molecular biological techniques to human neoplasms will certainly provide additional markers, but one caveat must be remembered as we look realistically towards the future: in a qualitative sense, no analyte has been associated with a human neoplasm that has not been shown to be present in a normal cell. It thus seems unlikely that absolute specificity for cancer will ever be realized.

ACID PHOSPHATASE

There is a long history of interest in the application of tumour markers to the prostate. Indeed, the first clinical use of *any* serum marker was the report of Gutman and Gutman[1], who measured acid phosphatase in men with prostatic carcinoma. Many studies have appeared since that time, using first enzymatic and later immunometric assays for initially non-specific, and subsequently prostate-specific, acid phosphatase. At one point it was even claimed that this test would serve as an equivalent to the cervical smear or the 'male Pap test'; with further research, it has been shown that owing to a lack of sensitivity to early-stage disease, this test has little or no role in diagnosis.

While formerly used widely, prostatic acid phosphatase (**Table 6.1**) has largely been replaced by

Table 6.1 Serum acid phosphatase vs. clinical stage						
	Assay type	Per cent abnormal by stage				
		OC	C	C&D	D	
Foti *et al.* (1977)[35]	E	14	29		60	
Cooper *et al.* (1978)[36]	E	9		46		
Bruce *et al.* (1980)[37]	E	9	17		73	
Murphy *et al.* (1979)[38]	E	11	17		51	
Van Cangh *et al.* (1982)[39]	E	21	31		78	
Foti *et al.* (1977)[35]	I	60	71		92	
Cooper *et al.* (1978)[36]	I	43		94		
Bruce *et al.* (1981)[40]	I	22	24		78	
Murphy *et al.* (1979)[38]	I	36	49		69	
Van Cangh *et al.* (1982)[39]	I	21	54		89	

E = Enzymatic assay, I = Immunologic assay
OC = Organ confined, D = Disseminated, C = Capsular penetration

prostate specific antigen (PSA) for clinical staging. Although a correlation occurs between the pathological stage and the serum acid phosphatase levels, a substantial overlap precludes any useful stratification. In addition, acid phosphatase is abnormal in only about two thirds of patients with organ-confined carcinoma. The one group where acid phosphatase remains useful, at least in the eyes of many investigators, is patients with clinically localized disease with an abnormal enzymatic acid phosphatase level[2]; this category, referred to as Mo (or Do) by some, has been shown to have an ominous prognosis, with clinical evidence of progression in the majority of patients in a relatively short time.

Recently, the group from Johns Hopkins University[3] has shown that it is unusual for acid phosphatase to provide unique information with respect to PSA in staging of prostatic carcinoma (less than 1% of patients). In general, there is now little justification for the primary-care provider or urologist to use this marker.

PROSTATE SPECIFIC ANTIGEN

Prostate specific antigen represents the best serum marker for prostatic carcinoma, and indeed could be argued to be the best tumour marker available today. It has established utilities both as an immunohistochem-

ical marker, and as a method of monitoring patients with established malignancy. The utility of PSA for staging and diagnosis, especially in the early-detection arena, is currently undergoing detailed investigation.

PSA is a 34 kilodalton glycoprotein, which is specific to prostatic epithelium (**6.1**). It is a neutral serine protease whose function is to lyse seminal-vesicle protein. Although most PSA remains within the prostatic ducts, a proportion is absorbed into the blood stream where to a large extent it is bound mainly to two proteins: anti-chymotrypsin (ACT) and alpha macroglobulin (**6.2**). Initial reports of a serum assay for PSA using simple electrophoresis[4] were insensitive, demonstrating elevated levels in only 17 out of 219 patients with prostatic carcinoma (8%). More sensitive assays were developed later.

Four commercial assays are readily available in the United States (**Table 6.2**) and many more in Europe; two by Hybritech Inc. (Hybritech Inc., San Diego, CA) make use of monoclonal technology. The Tandem-R and Tandem-E assays are different only in that the former is a radioimmunometric assay, while the latter is an immunoenzymatic assay. FDA approval has recently been granted for the Hybritech assay to be used for the early detection or screening of prostate cancer, in addition to its prior approval for monitoring. The Pros-check assay (Yang Laboratories, Bellevue, WA) is a conventional radioimmunoassay, utilizing polyclonal rabbit

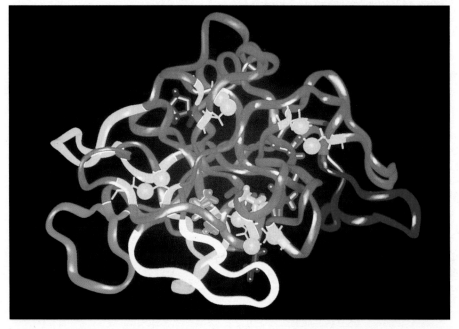

6.1 Three-dimensional molecular model of PSA (figure kindly supplied by Dominique P Bridon of Abbott Laboratories).

sera. Finally, Abbott Laboratories (Abbott Laboratories, Chicago, IL) has recently released the IMX PSA assay, employing a combination of monoclonal and polyclonal serum in an immunoradiometric format. A detailed discussion of the performance characteristics of these assays, as well as PSA in general, can be found in several recent reviews[5-7]. The use of PSA in early detection and screening is discussed in Chapter 7.

Early reports demonstrating that PSA was elevated in a proportion of patients with benign prostatic hyperplasia[8-11] (**Table 6.3**) in fact hindered interest in the use of PSA for the diagnosis of carcinoma. Because of the virtual certainty that men being evaluated for CaP would have at least histological BPH, it was reasoned that the specificity of an elevated PSA would be simply too low.

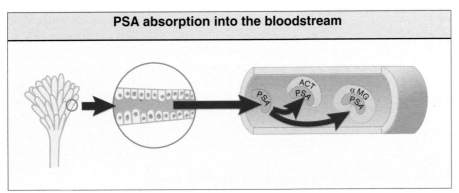

PSA absorption into the bloodstream

6.2 PSA is exclusively secreted from the epithelial cells of the prostatic ducts. A small proportion is absorbed into the blood stream where it is largely bound to either anti-chymotrypsin (ACT) or alpha macroglobulin (αMG), leaving only a small proportion of free, uncomplexed PSA.

Table 6.2 PSA assay comparison

	Tandem-R	Tandem-E	Pros-check	IMX
Assay Type	Immunoradiometric	Immunoenzymatic	Radioimmunoassay	Microparticle Enzyme Immunoassay
Assay Time	2 hours	4 hours	4.5 hr/ overnight	41 min.
Assay Range (ng/ml)	0–100	0–150	0–50	0–100
Antibodies	Monoclonal	Monoclonal	Polyclonal	Monoclonal/ Polyclonal
Normal Range (ng/ml)	0.0–4.0	0.0–4.0	0.0–2.5	0.0–4.0
Analytical Sensitivity (ng/ml)	0.1–0.2	0.1–0.2	0.1–0.2	< 0.1

PSA levels in prostatic fluid are approximately one million-fold higher than serum PSA values. An epithelial layer, a basal-cell layer, and a basement membrane separate the intraductal PSA from the capillary and lymphatic drainage of the prostate. Disruption of these barriers may allow increased PSA leakage into the interstitial tissue spaces and the systemic circulation resulting in elevated serum PSA levels (**6.3**).

The specificity for prostatic tissue of antibodies to PSA makes it a uniquely suitable marker for immuno-histochemically identifying prostate as the site of origin for poorly differentiated neoplasms of unknown aetiology. Primary and metastatic lesions almost invariably continue to express PSA, albeit in variable degrees, and the presence of PSA staining infers that the prostate is the site of origin. This may be exceedingly useful in cases of metastatic carcinoma of unknown origin (**6.4, Table 6.4**).

In attempts to further establish the relationship of serum PSA to the underlying prostate pathology, simple prostatectomy specimens were studied from 81 men with bladder outlet obstruction symptoms which were considered to be secondary to BPH[12]. In this study, pre-operative serum PSA was correlated with the pathology observed on histological section of all tissue removed. It was found that 36 of the 81 men (44%) had a PSA > 4.0 ng/ml. However, 35 had significant pathology which could allow leakage of PSA into the systemic circulation (**6.5**). This observation suggests that significant pathological lesions associated with disruption of the basal-cell layer, rather than the presence of BPH itself, explains the majority of elevations of serum PSA.

Several clinical parameters need to be considered when evaluating serum PSA levels. Brawer *et al.* reported that digital rectal examination was not associated

Table 6.3 Serum PSA in patients with histologically confirmed benign prostatic hyperplasia (%)			
Author	Assay	PSA >4.0 ng/ml	PSA>10.0 ng/ml
Ercole[41]	Tandem-R	75 (21)	10 (3)
Ferro[42]	Tandem-R		13 (33)
Hudson[43]	Tandem-R	35 (21)	3 (2)
Stamey[16]	Pros-check	70 (88)	

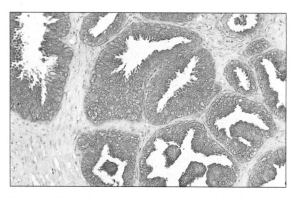

6.3 Anti-PSA staining showing strong positive (brown) staining of columnar epithelial cells of normal prostatic acini. (Reproduced from Weiss MA, Mills SE *Atlas of Genitourinary Tract Disorders* Gower, 1988.)

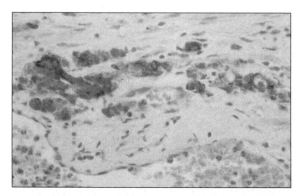

6.4 Immunohistochemical staining of PSA demonstrated in a poorly differentiated metastatic lesion from the prostate.

with erroneous elevation of PSA[13], and Crawford and associates[14] as well as Yuan et al.[15] confirm this.

More significant prostatic perturbations, such as prostate needle biopsy, urethral instrumentation and transurethral resection *will* cause significant elevation of serum PSA. Yuan and associates[15] noted that prostate needle biopsy resulted in a significant elevation of PSA that lasted for more than two weeks in 27 of 89 men. Brawer et al. studied 127 men following six-sector ultrasound-guided transrectal prostate needle biopsies, and noted a 20% or greater elevation in PSA levels 28 days after the procedure, when compared to prebiopsy level[7]. Patient age also has an effect on the PSA level; in a screening study of 1249 healthy men, PSA correlated significantly with patient age (**Table 6.5**). Oesterling has made similar observations (**6.6**).

Table 6.4 PSA immunohistochemistry

Author	Primary prostate cancer	Metastatic prostate cancer	Irradiated prostate cancer	Other tumours
Nadji et al.[44]	73/73	49/49		0/78
Stein et al.[45]	13/15			
Vernon and Williams[46]	30/30		5/5	
Ford et al.[47]	63/65	16/17		0/13
Brawer et al.[48]			33/33	
Sohlberg et al.[49]	23/23			
Total	202/206	65/66	38/38	0/91

Simple prostatectomy and PSA

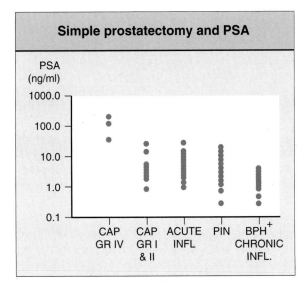

6.5 Pre-operative PSA values grouped for various pathologies identified at prostatectomy. Reproduced from Brawer et al. *Am J Clin Path* 1989;**92**(6):760–764.)

Table 6.5 Serum PSA versus age in screened population

Age (yrs)	PSA (ng/ml)			
	No. (%)	Mean	Median	SD
50–59	222 (17.8)	1.62	1.0	6.5
60–69	600 (48.0)	2.7	3.8	1.4
70–79	365 (29.2)	3.1	5.0	1.7
> 79	62 (5.0)	8.8	11.9	2.2
Total	1249	2.9	2.2	10.4

(Reproduced from Brawer et al. *J Urol* 1992;**147**: 841–845.)

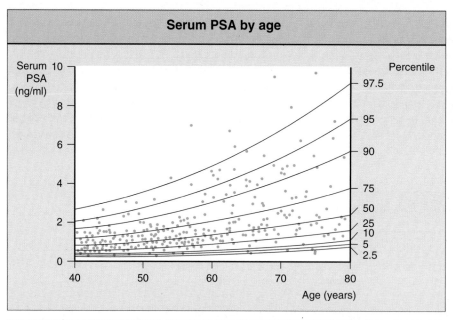

6.6 Serum PSA versus patient age in a cohort of patients without evidence of prostate cancer. (Modified with permission from Oesterling JE *et al. JAMA* 1993;**270**:840–864.)

Table 6.6 PSA and pathological stage

Author	Assay	PSA > 4.0 ng/ml				PSA > 10.0 ng/ml			
		OC	CP	SV	LN	OC	CP	SV	LN
Ercole et al.[41]	TANDEM-R	12 (40)	14 (74)	8 (100)	17 (100)	2 (7)	6 (32)	8 (100)	12 (71)
Hudson et al.[43]	TANDEM-R					3 (11)	5 (56)	0	2 (100)
Oesterling et al.[21]	TANDEM-R	47 (46)	26 (65)	13 (72)	17 (100)	10 (10)	8 (20)	11 (61)	12(71)
Stamey 13 (100) et al.[50]	PROSCHECK					NS	23 (82)	20 (95)	

OC = organ confined, CP = capsular penetration, SV = seminal vesicle involved, LN = node positive

PSA AND STAGING

PSA correlates with the clinical and, more reliably, the pathological stage of prostatic carcinoma (**Table 6.6**). Furthermore, the Stanford group correlated the volume of prostatic carcinoma with serum PSA level[16]; these authors demonstrated that each gram of prostatic carcinoma contributed around 3.5 ng/ml to the serum PSA level, and these data have been confirmed by others[17]. While there is a good correlation between the serum PSA level and the pathological stage in groups of patients, PSA is a relatively poor predictor of pathological stage for an individual patient[18] because of substantial overlap of PSA levels within any stage. PSA values vary widely among disease stage, and overlapping of stages further confounds the predictive value of PSA to pathological stage.

As mentioned earlier, PSA values can be greatly affected by any invasive prostatic manipulation. For this reason, prebiopsy PSA values are much better correlated to pathological stage than are postbiopsy PSA values. In our study, where PSA determinations were carried out prior to significant prostatic perturbation and then radical prostatectomy was performed, none of the fourteen tumours found in men with prebiopsy values greater than 10.0 ng/ml was organ-confined on pathological examination. A recent study by the Washington University group confirms these observations[19]. In this study, 14 out of 16 patients with biopsy-proven prostate carcinoma and a serum PSA of greater than 10.0 ng/ml were found to have extracapsular disease. These observations suggest that a good correlation exists between serum PSA values of greater than 10.0 ng/ml by the Hybritech method and the presence of extracapsular tumour extension.

Serum PSA values have also proven useful in the determination of bone metastases in untreated prostate cancer patients. The Mayo Clinic group[20] found that only 1 of 306 patients with serum PSA values of less than 20 ng/ml (Tandem-R) had a positive bone scan. The probability of a positive bone scan with a serum PSA of 10.0 ng/ml or less was estimated at 1.4%. PSA was found to be a more reliable and accurate indicator of bony metastases than clinical stage, tumour grade, acid phosphates, or PAP. It should be noted, however, that only 7 of the 852 men studied actually had a positive bone scan. Of course, any patient with skeletal pain should be fully staged by radionucleoide bone scan, but the need for cost savings may lead to a more selective approach to ordering bone scans in asymptomatic men and during follow-up.

PSA AFTER RADICAL PROSTATECTOMY

Within a few weeks following a radical prostatectomy with negative surgical margins, the serum PSA should theoretically be zero; this level should be attained within 3–4 weeks post-operatively[21] as the half-life of PSA is between 2.2 and 3.2 days. Unfortunately, none of the currently available assays for PSA can measure levels down to zero. The biological sensitivity of the assay (that level of serum PSA which can be distinguished from zero with 95% certainty) varies between commercial assays, and must be determined in an individual laboratory by repetitive testing.

After radical prostatectomy or radiotherapy, serum PSA is generally the first indicator of 'recurrent' disease. Carter et al.[22] noted that no patient with undetectable PSA level after radical prostatectomy had clinical evidence of active prostate cancer. Carter further noted that all patients with clinically detectable distant recurrences had elevated PSA post-operatively. Stamey et al.[16] added to these findings by noting that no patients who failed to normalize serum PSA within

3 weeks of radical prostatectomy had a subsequent decrease in PSA levels to undetectable range without adjuvant therapy.

Several studies imply that the majority of patients with undetectable PSA values following radical prostatectomy will remain without evidence of recurrence, whereas those whose PSA levels remain detectable will almost always experience some type of recurrence. Lange et al.[23] measured PSA levels three to six months after radical prostatectomy and correlated the results with clinical outcome: in men with PSA levels ≤ 0.2 ng/ml, only 11% recurred; for those who had PSA > 0.4 ng/ml, 100% recurred. In following 86 patients who had undetectable PSA levels after radical prostatectomy, seven (8.1%) had a subsequent rise in PSA levels to a mean of 70.6 ng/ml. Stein et al.[24] reported that in all cases of a group of 230 patients with pathological stage T1–T2, non-metastatic disease followed for a mean of 48 months after radical retropubic prostatectomy; elevations of serum PSA preceded the clinical recurrence of disease. However, in 41 out of 175 patients with detectable PSA values and no clinical evidence of recurrent prostate cancer, elevated serum PSA levels suggested a recurrence. The 5-year and 10-year clinical disease-free survivals were 82% and 72% respectively. If an elevated serum PSA value was taken to indicate recurrent disease, then the 5-year and 10-year disease-free survival decreases to 62% and 41% respectively. Thus, even 10 years after radical prostatectomy, a significant percentage of patients with apparent, recurrent, prostate cancer by biochemical parameters remain without other clinical evidence of the disease.

Detecting the location of low-volume, persistent disease can be difficult. Digital rectal examinations are often inconclusive, and bone scan and computerized tomography scan are generally negative in these patients. Lightner and associates[25], in evaluating needle biopsy of the anastomosis (NBA) in a group of men with serum PSA value >0.4 ng/ml after radical prostatectomy, found that 42% of the patients had a positive needle biopsy but negative bone scans and CT scans. No patient with a nondetectable PSA value had a positive needle biopsy of the anastomosis. Foster et al.[26] and Abi-Aad and associates[27] observed similar findings, reporting positive biopsies among 45% and 40%, respectively of those patients with elevated PSA values following radical prostatectomy.

The development of more sensitive assays for PSA should allow earlier detection of persistent disease[28]. Takayama et al.[29] found a 9–12 month lead time in detecting persistent disease using 0.1 ng/ml rather than 0.4 ng/ml of serum PSA to indicate persistent disease. All patients in this group whose serum PSA reached a level of 0.1 ng/ml continued to show a rise in PSA levels. No patient who had a serum PSA value <0.1 ng/ml at 36 months after radical prostatectomy developed recurrent disease; the Stanford group[30] has reported similar findings.

Whether the early treatment of patients with biochemical evidence of recurrent disease will result in prolonged survival remains to be determined.

There is some evidence indicating that patients who fail to normalize their PSA initially are more likely to have distant metastases, while those who develop delayed PSA elevations after radical prostatectomy more often have a local recurrence. Lange et al.[23] treated 29 patients who had elevated PSA values and negative CT scans and bone scans with pelvic irradiation. PSA values decreased by more than 50% in 82% of the patients. Forty-three percent of the patients had an accompanying decrease in serum PSA within six months, to an undetectable range. Link et al.[8] reported similar findings in an evaluation of 2 groups of patients with adjuvant radiation therapy. They found that only 1 out of 12 patients (8%) receiving radiation treatment for elevated PSA immediately after prostatectomy, versus 7 of 15 (54%) patients receiving radiation treatment for a delayed elevation in PSA after radical prostatectomy, had continued suppression of PSA levels at undetectable levels during an average 33 month follow-up.

PSA AFTER RADIATION THERAPY

PSA also offers new information on the behaviour of prostate cancer following radiation therapy. Serum PSA has been found to decrease following radiation therapy, with a half life estimated at between 1.4 and 2.6 months[9,10]. The Stanford group[11] followed 183 patients after completion of radiation therapy (most of whom had localized disease) for a mean of 61 months. Serum PSA was reduced to undetectable levels in 11% of the patients; 25% of patients had a decrease in serum PSA values to the normal range (less than 2.5 ng/ml, Pros-check). Elevated PSA levels persisted in 65% of patients. Radiation therapy during the first year caused a reduction in PSA values in 82% of patients. Continued reduction after the first year of therapy occurred in only 8% of patients. PSA values rose in 51% of the patients.

Russell et al.[31] reported that pretreatment PSA values are associated with the chance of complete response (normalization of PSA with no tumour detectable by radiographic studies or digital rectal examination). In an evaluation of 143 men who were treated with external-beam irradiation (either photon or fast neutron) for clinically localized prostate cancer with a median follow-up of 27 months, patients with a pretreatment PSA value that was less than 4 times the normal had an 82% chance of complete response. Those with a PSA value greater than 4 times the normal value were associated with only a 30% chance of complete response. Furthermore, the time to normalization of PSA also appears to be important. In Russell and colleagues' study, 94% of those with normalization of PSA within 6 months remained complete responders during the study, compared with 8% of men with persistently elevated PSA values after 6 months.

Meek and associates[9] conducted a similar study of serum PSA and radiotherapy for prostate cancer. They found a post-treatment PSA nadir in the normal range to be the most important prognostic variable. Pretreatment PSA was not predictive of outcome if serum prostatic acid phosphates (PAPs) were considered. They also noted that the initial rate of PSA decrease was unrelated to outcome.

Kabalin[12] conducted transrectal ultrasound-guided sextant biopsies on 27 men 18 months after external-beam radiation therapy. Persistent prostate carcinoma was detected in 25 of the 27 patients, including 20 of 22 men in whom it was also detectable with normal digital rectal examination. All four patients with normal PSA levels (<2.5 ng/ml, Pros-check), including one patient with an undetectable PSA, had positive biopsies. This suggests that rising PSA levels after radiation therapy do in fact indicate persistent disease. Such rises should prompt further evaluation with prostate needle biopsy if the patient is a candidate for salvage radical prostatectomy.

PSA AND HORMONAL THERAPY

The PSA nadir also appears to be an important indicator of response to hormonal therapy. Stamey et al.[32] followed a cohort of patients with metastatic prostate cancer after initiation of hormonal therapy. Twenty-two percent of the patients had a decrease in serum PSA levels to the normal range, while 9% had a decrease to undetectable levels. Of 11 patients who were followed with frequent PSA determinations following the induction of hormonal therapy, the PSA nadir was reached within 5 months in 9 of the 11. Seventy-two percent of the patients were noted to have increasing PSA values after 6 months. The effect of hormonal ablation on serum PSA is extremely variable.

Miller et al.[33] studied serum PSA levels of 48 patients with metastatic prostate cancer who achieved an objective response to hormonal therapy. They found that patients who reached a PSA nadir of less than 4.0 ng/ml had a significantly longer duration of remission than those who failed to normalize their PSA levels. No patient gave evidence of progressive disease while the PSA level was decreasing or at the nadir level. They also noted that a rise in serum PSA predated other evidence of disease progression by a mean of 7.3 months. Gillatt et al.[34] also reported that PSA levels are significantly related to survival after initiation of hormonal therapy in his study of 136 men with metastatic prostate cancer whose PSA levels were determined at 3 and 6 months following therapy initiation.

SUMMARY

PSA is arguably the most valuable tumour marker available in all oncology. This analyte can be successfully used to diagnose, stage and monitor prostatic carcinoma. Refinement of PSA assays continues to contribute to their clinical use and allows for earlier detection of persistent disease after radical surgery. While there have been significant advances in the use of PSA as a tumour marker, shortcomings exist, and the measure continues to be controversial in prostate cancer screening. Further evaluation of new ideas such as PSA density and annualized PSA 'velocity' or 'slope' seem likely to contribute to our knowledge of PSA and its clinical applications.

REFERENCES

1. Gutman AB, Gutman EB. 'Acid' phosphatase activity of the serum of normal human subjects. Proc Soc Exp Biol Med 1938;38:470.
2. Whitesel J, Donohue R, Mani J et al. Acid phosphatase: Its influence on the management of carcinoma of the prostate. J Urol 1984;131:70–72.
3. Burnett AL, Chan DW, Brendler CB, et al. Is it necessary to measure serum enzymatic acid phosphatase prior to radical prostatectomy [Abstract]? J Urol 1992;147:361.
4. Papsidero L et al. A prostate antigen in sera of prostatic cancer patients. Cancer Res 1980;40:2428–2432.
5. Brawer MK, Lange PH. Prostate specific antigen: Its role in early detection, staging and monitoring of prostatic carcinoma. Endourology 1989;3(2):227–236.
6. Oesterling J. Prostate specific antigen: a critical assessment of the most useful tumor marker for adenocarcinoma of the prostate. J Urol 1991;145:907–923.
7. Ellis WJ, Brawer MK. 'The role of tumor markers in the diagnosis and treatment of prostate cancer.' in Prostate Diseases. Lepor (ed.) 1993, W.B. Saunders. Philadelphia.
8. Link P, Freiha F, Stamey T. Adjuvant radiation therapy in patients with detectable prostate specific antigen following radical prostatectomy. J Urol 1991;145:532–534.
9. Meek AG, Park TL, Oberman E, et al. A prospective study of PSA levels in patients receiving radiotherapy for localized carcinoma of the prostate. Int J Radiat Oncol Biol Phys 1990;75:1982.
10. Ritter MA, Messing EM, Shanahan TG, et al. Prostate-specific antigen as a predictor of radiotherapy response and patterns of failure in localized prostate cancer. J Clin Oncol 1992;10:1208–1217.
11. Stamey TA, Kabalin JN, Ferrari M. Prostate specific antigen in the diagnosis and treatment of adenocarcinoma of the prostate. III. Radiation treated patients. J Urol 1989;141:1083–1087.
12. Kabalin J, Hodge K, McNeal J, et al. Identification of residual cancer in the prostate following radiation therapy: Role of transrectal ultrasound guided biopsy and prostate specific antigen. JUrol 1989;142:326.
13. Brawer M, Schifman R, Ahmann F, et al. The effect of digital rectal examination on serum levels of prostatic-specific antigen. Arch Pathol Lab Med 1988;112:1110.
14. Crawford E, Schutz M, drago J, et al. The effect of digital rectal examination on PSA. J Urol 1991;145:398A.
15. Yuan JJ, Catalona WJ. Effect of digital rectal examination, prostate massage, transrectal ultrasonography and needle biopsy of the prostate on serum prostate specific antigen levels. J Urol 1991;145: 213A.
16. Stamey TA, Yang N, Hay AR. et al. Prostate-specific antigen as a serum marker for adenocarcinoma of the prostate. N Engl J Med 1987;317:909–916.
17. Partin A, Carter H, Chan D, et al. Prostate specific antigen in the staging of localized prostate cancer: Influence of tumor differentiation, tumor volume and benign hyperplasia. J Urol 1990;143:747–752.
18. Brawer MK, Lange PH. Prostate specific antigen in management of prostatic carcinoma. Suppl to Urol 1989;33:11.
19. Catalona W, Smith D, Ratcliff T, et al.. Measurement of prostate-specific antigen in serum as a screening test for prostate cancer. N. Engl. J Med. 1991;324:1156–1161.

20. Oesterling JE, Martin SK, Bergstraih EJ, et al. The use of prostate-specific antigen in staging patients with newly diagnosed prostate cancer. JAMA 1993;**269(1)**:57–60.

21. Oesterling J, Chan D, Epstein J, et al.. Prostate specific antigen in the preoperative and postoperative evaluation of localized prostatic cancer treated with radical prostatectomy. J Urol 1988;**139**:766–772.

22. Carter HB, Partin AW, Oesterling JE, et al. The use of PSA in the management of patients with prostate cancer: The Johns Hopkins experience. Clinical Aspects of Prostate Cancer 1989;247–254.

23. Lange PH, Lightner DJ, Medini E, et al. The effect of radiation therapy after radical prostatectomy in patients with elevated PSA levels. J Urol 1990;**144**: 927.

24. Stein A, deKernion JB, Smith RB, Dorey F and Patel H. PSA levels after radical prostatectomy in patients with organ confined and locally extensive prostate cancer. J Urol 1992;**147**:942.

25. Lightner D, Lange P, Reddy P, et al. Prostate specific antigen and local recurrence after radical prostatectomy. J Urol. 1990;**144**:921.

26. Foster LS, Shinahara K, Carol P, et al. The value of PSA and transrectal ultrasound-guided biopsy in accurately detecting prostatic fossa recurrences following radical prostatectomy. J Urol 1993;**149**:1024.

27. Abi-Aad AS, Macfarlane MT, Stein A et al. Detection of local recurrence after radical prostatectomy by PSA and TRUS. J Urol. 1992;**147**:952.

28. Vessella RL, Noteboom J, Lange PH. Evaluation of the Abbott IMX (R) automated immunoassay of PSA. Clin Chem. 1992;**38**:2044.

29. Takayama TK, Vessella RL, Brawer MK, et al. The enhanced detection of persistent disease after radical prostatectomy with a new PSA immunoassay. J Urol. 1993;**150**:374.

30. Stamey TA, Graves H, Wehner N, et al. Early Detection of Residual Prostate Cancer after Radical Prostatectomy by an Ultrasensitive Assay for Prostate Specific Antigen. J Urol 1993;**149**:787–792.

31. Russell KJ, Dunatov C, Hafermann JT, et al.. Prostate specific antigen in the management of patients with localized andenocarcinoma of the prostate treated with primary radiation therapy. J Urol 1991;**146**:1041–1052.

32. Stamey TA, Kabalin JN, Ferrari M, et al. Prostate specific antigen in the diagnosis and treatment of adenocarcinoma of the prostate: IV. Anti-androgen treated patients. J Urol. 1989;**141**:1088–1090.

33. Miller JI, Ahman FR, Drach GW, et al.. The clinical usefulness of serum PSA after hormonal therapy of metastatic prostate cancer. J Urol. 1992;**147**:956.

34. Gillatt D, Gingell C and Smith PJB. Serum PSA for the assessment of response to hormonal therapy. J Urol. 1990;**143**: 207A.

35. Foti AG, Cooper JF, Herschman H, et al. Detection of prostatic cancer by solid-phase radioimmunoassay of serum prostatic acid phosphatase. N Engl J Med. 1977;**297**:1357–1361.

36. Cooper JF, Foti AG, Herschman HH, et al.. A solid phase-radioimmunoassay for prostatic acid phosphatase. J Urol. 1978;**119**:388.

37. Bruce AW, Mahan DE, Belville WD. The role of the radioimmunoassay for prostatic acid phosphatase in prostatic carcinoma. Urol Clin N Amer. 1980;**7**:645.

38. Murphy GP, Chu TM, Karr JP. Prostatic acid phosphatase – the developing experience. Clin Biochem. 1979;**12**:226.

39. Van Cangh PJ, Opsomer R, de Nayer P. Serum prostatic acid phosphatase determination in prostatic diseases: a critical comparison of an enzymatic and a radioimmunologic assay. J Urol 1982;**128**:1212.

40. Bruce A, Mahan D, Sullivan L, et al. The significance of prostatic acid phosphatase and adenocarcinoma of the prostate. J Urol 1981;**125**:357.

41. Ercole C, Lange P, Mathisen M, et al. Prostate specific antigen and prostatic acid phosphatase in the monitoring and staging of patients with prostatic cancer. J Urol. 1987;**138**:1181–1184.

42. Ferro M, Barnes I, Roberts J, et al. Tumor markers in prostatic carcinoma. A comparison of prostate-specific antigen with acid phosphatase. Br J Urol 1987;**60**:69.

43. Hudson M, Bahnson R, Catalona W. Clinical use of prostate specific antigen in patients with prostate cancer. J Urol 1989;**142**:1011.

44. Nadji M, Tabei S, Castro A, et al. Prostatic-specific antigen: An immunohistologic marker for prostatic neoplasms. Cancer 1981;**48**:1229–1232.

45. Stein BS, Petersen RO, Vangore S, et al. Immunoperoxidase localization of PSA. Am J Surg Path 1982;**6**:553.

46. Vernon S, Williams W. Pre-treatment and post-treatment evaluation of prostatic adenocarcinoma for prostatic specific acid phosphatase and prostatic specific antigen by immunohistochemistry. J Urol 1983;**130**: 95–98.

47. Ford T, Butcher D, Masters J, et al. Immunocytochemical localization of prostate-specific antigen: specificity and application to clinical practice. Br J Urol 1985;**57**:50.

48. Brawer M, Nagle R, Pitts W, et al. Keratin immunoreactivity as an aid to the diagnosis of persistent adenocarcinoma in irradiated human prostates. Cancer 1989;**63**:454.

49. Sohlberg OE, Bigler SA, Brawer MK. PSA immunohistochemistry in PIN. J Urol 1990;**143**:202A.

50. Stamey TA, Kabalin JN. Prostate specific antigen in the diagnosis and treatment of adenocarcinoma of the prostate: I. Untreated patients. J. Urol 1989;**141**:1070–1075.

CHAPTER 7

SCREENING FOR
PROSTATE CANCER

INTRODUCTION

In the United States especially, both the general interest in prostatic carcinoma and the early detection/screening for this common neoplasm have already achieved staggering levels. The recent recommendations by the American Cancer Society[1], as well as the American Urologic Association, of an annual DRE and PSA test for all men over 50 for early detection of prostate cancer has further fostered interest in this area. The rest of the world has watched with some bemusement the machinations of urologists, oncologists, and primary-care practitioners, along with health planners, economists and the lay press in the US wrestling with the complex issues of early detection and screening. The need to resolve these conflicts for the sake of the patients has prompted both European and US randomized studies in screening for this most prevalent of neoplasms in men beyond middle age.

Despite a very real increase in the depth of our knowledge of prostatic carcinoma, which ranges from epidemiological insight into the perplexing increase in both incidence and mortality from this cancer, to our increasing understanding of the molecular basis of the disease, therapeutic advances, and improvement in diagnostic technology – the *sine qua non* of any screening protocol, proof that cancer-related mortality can be decreased – has not yet been achieved.

This has led many to assume a negative if not nihilistic attitude towards early detection. However, one is sobered by the reality that prostatic cancer is the number one malignancy in incidence in US men, and the second most common cause of cancer-related death[2,3]. Moreover, it is estimated that in the USA by the end of the century there will have been a 37% increase in the rate of prostate cancer deaths, and a 90% increase in diagnoses compared with the early 1980s[4].

It is clearly not feasible to wait 10–15 years, when the efficacy of early detection and treatment may be provided by the several international studies currently underway. Urologists worldwide must at least understand the lessons to be gleaned from the *existing* data, and apply this information wisely in order to help their patients make informed and rational decisions when faced with this insidious, and often lethal, disease.

It may sometimes be difficult to distinguish between screening and early detection. In the broad sense, *screening* represents the physician-initiated search for disease by invitation in an asymptomatic subject, and is distinct from *early detection*, which attempts to identify a condition in patients seeking medical care – albeit for an unrelated malady. From an epidemiological and ethical perspective these are certainly separable. However, by the time a patient presents to a clinician, the differences pale and the physician is in fact involved in early detection.

Historically, we have observed that the clinical diagnosis of prostate cancer is insensitive for identifying men with curable malignancies. Approximately 30% of patients present with disseminated disease with a median duration of survival of less than three years[5–8], and 30% of patients have clinical evidence of tumour extension beyond the confines of the prostate at the time of presentation[9,10]. Among such men, irrespective of the therapeutic approach employed, evidence of disease progression occurs generally within 10 years[9,11,12].

Thus, if clinical parameters are relied upon, only approximately 40% of patients have potentially curable malignancy at the time of presentation. Of these, 10% have minimal cancer which is found upon simple prostatectomy, and which most clinicians believe does not require aggressive management. Therefore, without screening, less than one-third of all men presenting with carcinoma are suitable candidates for curative therapy. Among this third, pathological upstaging at radical prostatectomy occurs in approximately half[9,5,13,10].

Currently, therefore, only about 15% of those presenting clinically with prostate cancer have potentially curable neoplasm. Even among these most favourable patients, significant cancer-related mortality occurs, even with aggressive radiation therapy[14,15] or radical prostatectomy[16-18]. It is therefore clear that routine clinical approaches to the identification of men with prostate cancer are woefully inadequate. Most patients present with advanced local or metastatic disease, and even among those with favourable clinical parameters, cancer progression with its long, drawn-out morbidity and negative effects on the quality of life occurs all too often.

Prostate cancer clearly represents a significant problem. How, then, can we decrease cancer-related mortality? In general, for all neoplasms, we have three options: we can prevent the incidence of the disease; we can improve curative therapy; or we may increase early detection – that is, identify more patients with cancers amenable to cure (**Table 7.1**). We do not know what causes prostate cancer, and until we do it is unlikely that we can significantly reduce the incidence. A large-scale chemoprevention trial utilizing the 5-alpha reductase finasteride is currently underway in the USA, and other chemopreventative approaches are being considered. These investigations may result in a decrease in the incidence of prostate cancer, but the data will not be forthcoming for many years.

The second option in the battle to reduce prostate cancer-related mortality is to improve the efficacy of therapy. This is discussed in subsequent chapters on treatment. Suffice it to say here that while significant strides have been made in decreasing the morbidity of radiation therapy, radical prostatectomy as well as hormonal manipulation, whether any of these approaches has truly decreased cancer-related mortality remains to be proven. Thus we are left with early detection or screening in an attempt to reduce the death rate from

this cancer. If treatment for localized carcinoma is indeed effective, then identification of a greater percentage of men with early disease makes intuitive sense. The widespread application of the early detection of prostate cancer stems from this logic.

For early detection, or indeed screening, to make sense, the disease in question must fulfil a number of criteria (**Table 7.2**). First, it should have a high prevalence; in a disease with a low prevalence, too many subjects must be tested for each carcinoma found, resulting in significant logistic as well as economic problems. Certainly prostatic carcinoma fulfills the requirement of high prevalence. Confounding this, however, is a unique feature of prostate cancer: the fact that the autopsy prevalence far exceeds that of clinically manifest disease. As previously cited, approximately 30% of men undergoing post-mortem examination without a clinical history of prostate cancer can be demonstrated to have histological evidence of prostatic cancer on serial sections of their prostate[16-19]. Cystoprostatectomy specimens from men with transitional-cell carcinoma of the urinary bladder have confirmed these findings[20-23]. For example, in 1985, 86 000 diagnoses of prostatic carcinoma were made in the United States. This represented only 1.05% of the estimated 8 193 000 men with 'autopsy' or latent carcinoma. Thus, in 1985, 0.31% of those who we can assume had microscopic foci of prostate cancer actually died of the disease[24]. However, these data do not take into consideration the importance of the prolonged period of risk in a man's life for either cancer development or progression. Scardino[24] 'factored in' the important variable of time and concluded that the lifetime risk of developing 'autopsy cancer' was 42%; the lifetime risk of developing 'clinical cancer' based on data from Seidman[3] was 9.5%, and the lifetime risk of dying of prostatic carcinoma was 2.9%.

Table 7.1 Approaches to reduce cancer-related mortality

- Decrease incidence
- Improve therapy
- Provide early detection

Table 7.2 Screening essentials

- Significant disease
- Known natural history
- Effective therapy
- Availability of diagnostic tests
- Subject acceptance
- Cost effectiveness

The second requirement for an early detection or screening regimen is that the natural history of the disease be known. For prostate cancer, this is inextricably related to the dilemma associated with the discrepancy between histological evidence of disease and cancer-related morbidity and mortality. Of all human malignancies, prostate cancer exhibits the greatest variability in natural history, and it is in this arena that our ignorance makes recommendations about screening most troublesome.

A number of institutions have reported on the natural history of untreated prostatic carcinomas[25-30] (see **Table 7.3**). While one may derive information from these studies with respect to the outcome of untreated prostate cancer, the reader must be cautioned that all are hampered by methodological constraints; no report derives from a randomized controlled trial. Clearly, given the prevalence, we do not want to identify in early detection or screening programmes all of the men with cancers in their prostates. One might ask how many should be diagnosed? That is, how many cancers in men must we identify in order to offer treatment to the majority of patients whose malignancies would go on to affect the quantity or quality of their lives? While no definitive answer can be provided, Scardino and associates in a review of the features separating cancers with and without likely clinical sequelae have concluded that optimal efficiency would result if we could identify approximately 20% of the men with prostate cancer[31]. Thus, 6% (20% of the 30% autopsy prevalence) of men subjected to early detection/screening should have a cancer diagnosis. In the USA currently, it is estimated that around 3% of men will die eventually of prostate cancer. Implicit in this is the assurance that we can identify those cancers which possess a lethal potential during the course of the individual patient's lifetime, and successfully intervene. Moreover, we must not detect those much more prevalent malignancies that have low malignant potential. This is the most important issue in the early detection of prostatic carcinoma, and has already been discussed in the chapters on pathology and basic science issues.

The yield of any diagnostic test for detecting carcinoma obviously depends upon the prevalence of the disease in the population being evaluated. Because of variable study populations (i.e. whether patients present in a screening or early detection trial, are referred from other clinicians, or are gleaned from a urological practice) the prevalence of carcinoma may vary significantly; thus, meaningful comparison of studies of prostate cancer diagnosis is almost impossible. This must be remembered as we begin to examine the efficacy of screening tests.

Another essential for screening is the availability of diagnostic tests for the disease in question. In a sense, the elucidation of symptoms may be considered a test. Constitutional symptoms such as bone pain, weakness, weight loss, anaemia and uraemia may prompt the clinician to consider prostate carcinoma in the older man. Certainly such patients do not comprise an early detection or screening population. Symptomatic patients do, however, constitute a potential bias in the evaluation of the efficacy of early detection, because such patients generally have advanced disease. Comparison of the outcomes of those who present with symptoms, with those of healthy subjects participating in screening trials, almost universally results in the latter performing better. In general, neoplasms detected by screening are of smaller volume, lower

Table 7.3. Results of expectant management of prostatic carcinoma

Author	Number of patients	Mean F.U. (years)	Overall mortality (%)	CaP mortality (%)	CaP progression (includes CaP death)
Johansson[25]	223	10.2	56	8	34
Whitmore[26]	75	9.5	39	15	69
Hanash[27]	179	15	55	45	NA
George[28]	120	15	44	4	83
Madsen[29]	50	10	52	6	18

stage, and better differentiated than carcinomas that give rise to symptoms. This phenomenon constitutes the so-called 'length–time' bias (**Table 7.4**).

The most widely utilized test for the detection of prostate cancer is the digital rectal examination (DRE). The subjectivity of the DRE, differing skills among examiners and our increasing suspicion of subtle abnormalities, have resulted in great variability in the yield of cancer detected in men with an abnormality on digital rectal examination. Detection rates of 0.8–25.2% have been reported, along with positive predictive values of 6.3–50% (see **Table 7.5**).

In a series at the University of Washington, Seattle, carcinoma has been detected in 40 of 229 men (17.5%) with normal-feeling prostates undergoing biopsy because of elevated prostate specific antigen level, or being evaluated for alternative therapies to bladder-outlet obstruction owing to presumed BPH (**Table 7.6**). Twenty-four of 185 men (13.0%) with asymmetry as their only abnormality and 112 of 456 (24.6%) with prostatic induration revealed carcinoma. In contrast, 79 of 150 men (52.7%) with clearly palpable nodules or areas of marked induration strongly suggestive of carcinoma actually demonstrated malignancy.

Transrectal ultrasound (TRUS) is the most common approach for imaging the prostate; it offers several advantages to other imaging modalities. TRUS is a readily accepted, fairly simple procedure affording excellent visualization of the gland. It has the advantage of being able to identify suspicious lesions in the prostate which are non-palpable. A number of authorities, including Cooner et al.[32], Lee et al.[33] and Drago et al.[34], reported a 1.3–2 fold increase in the detection rate of carcinoma when digital rectal examination was compared to TRUS (**Table 7.7**). In early detection and screening studies, detection rates of 1.7–37.5%, and

Table 7.4 Length time bias

'Screened' patients	'Clinical' patients
Asymptomatic	Symptomatic
Earlier cancer	More advanced cancer
Slower growing	Rapidly growing
Lower stage	Higher stage
Lower grade	Higher grade

Table 7.5 Results of prostate cancer screening by digital rectal examination.

Source	No. of cancer/ no. of patients screened (%)	Positive predictive value
Catalona[54]	146/6630 (2.2)	146/683 (21.4)
Cooner[32]	203/807 (25.2)	203/470 (43.2)
Chodak[55]	36/2131 (1.7)	36/144 (25.0)
Faul[56]	1951/1,500,000 (0.1)	1951/11,308 (17.3)
Gilbertsen[57]	75/5856 (1.3)	–
Jenson[58]	36/4367 (0.8)	–
Lee[59]	10/784 (1.3)	10/29 (34.5)
McWhorter[60]	4/34 (1.8)	4/8 (50.0)
Mettlin[61]	33/2425 (13.6)	33/118 (28.0)
Mueller[62]	312/11,523 (2.7)	122/312 (39.1)
Thompson[63]	17/2005 (0.8)	17/65 (26.2)
Vihko[64]	6/771 (0.8)	6/27 (22.2)
Waaler[65]	1/480 (0.2)	1/16 (6.3)

positive predictive values of 6.8–58.3%, have been reported. However, the procedure is hampered by its high cost, and this, in conjunction with overall inadequate performance (sensitivity and specificity), makes this test unsuitable for the early detection of carcinoma. Despite these limitations, transrectal ultrasound-guided prostate needle biopsy employing the spring-loaded biopsy device is undoubtedly the best way of providing histological samples of the prostate. The procedure is simple and rapid with low, acceptable morbidity (around 2–3% infective complications) presuming that appropriate antimicrobial prophylaxis is administered.

Table 7.6 Yield for DRE in which all men underwent TRUS biopsy irrespective of the DRE result

DRE	Biopsy	Carcinoma (%)
Normal	224	40 (17.9)
Asymmetry	181	24 (13.3)
Induration	448	111 (24.8)
Malignant	148	78 (56.7)

Table 7.7 Results of prostate cancer screening by transrectal ultrasound

Author	No. of Cancer/ No. of Subjects Screened (%)	Positive Predictive Value (%)
Cooner[32]	263/1807 (14.6)	263/835 (31.5)
Devonec[66]	42/213 (19.7)	42/132 (31.8)
Fritzsche[67]	41/228 (18.0)	41/121 (33.9)
Hunter[68]	29/508 (5.7)	29/119 (24.4)
Lee[33]	20/748 (2.7)	20/64 (31.3)
McWhorter[60]	7/34 (20.6)	7/12 (58.3)
Mettlin[61]	44/2425 (1.8)	44/290 (15.2)
Perrin[69]	11/666 (1.7)	11/162 (6.8)
Ragde[70]	50/765 (6.5)	50/138 (36.2)
Rifkin[71]	3/112 (2.7)	3/8 (37.5)

Prostate specific antigen (PSA) has already been reviewed in Chapter 6. Here we shall confine our comments to its utility in early detection and screening. After the development of sensitive assays for serum PSA detection, considerable enthusiasm was generated for the utility of this test for the detection of prostate cancer. Several investigators have utilized PSA as the initial test in an early-detection programme. Catalona and associates[35], employing the Hybritech Tandem-R assay and utilizing a 4.0 ng/ml cut off, examined 1653 men over the age of 50. The overall detection rate was 2.2% and positive predictive value 33%.

At the University of Washington, Seattle, Brawer et al. have conducted a similar study examining 1249 men over age 50 with the Hybritech Tandem-R assay as the initial test in an early-detection programme[36]. The overall detection rate was 2.6% and the positive predictive value 30.5%. Two smaller screening studies in the UK also reported a detection rate of around 2%[37,38].

In an effort to understand how we should follow-up men with an initially normal PSA, Brawer et al. elected to perform digital rectal examination and transrectal ultrasound, as well as ultrasound-guided biopsy, in men in the original screening cohort who, on evaluation one year later, had a 20% increase in their PSA level[39]. Recently, Schmid and associates[40] demonstrated that the PSA doubling time in untreated localized prostate cancer is around 4–5 years, offering some biological rationale to our selection of a 20% cut off to select subjects for biopsy.

Seven hundred and one patients returned for the second year of our screening study. Two hundred and sixty (37.1%) demonstrated a greater than 20% increase in PSA value (**Table 7.8**). Biopsies were performed on 82 of these men and carcinoma detected in 14 (17.1%). Twelve of the men with carcinoma (86%) had a second year PSA <4.0 ng/ml. Radical prostatectomy was performed on 8 patients. Seven of these had organ-confined disease or tumour penetrating the capsule with negative surgical margins[39].

At Seattle we have recently completed the third year of studying the original cohort. Seven hundred and thirty eight men returned; 260 (35.2%) had a 20% annualized PSA elevation, 70 (50.8%) underwent biopsy, and carcinoma was detected in 13 (18.6%). The observed prostatic carcinoma detection rates for years 1–3 were 2.6, 2.0 and 1.8% respectively.

Despite the reasonable performance of PSA in an early-detection realm, one caveat must be noted. A significant number of men in whom prostatic carcinoma is detected have PSA < 4.0 ng/ml. For instance, in a recent compilation of our ultrasound-guided prostate needle biopsy series, carcinoma was noted in 256 of 1023 men (25.0%) who had undergone six systematic random biopsies. Fifty-three of these 256 patients (20.7%) had a pre-operative PSA level <4.0 ng/ml by the Hybritech Tandem method.

Comparison of these three diagnostic tests may be best achieved using the receiver-operating characteristic curve. When we applied this to our series at the University of Washington, PSA had the best performance characteristics (**7.1**).

A number of investigators have examined PSA in conjunction with other diagnostic techniques, primarily DRE and TRUS. Most studies have confirmed that approximately one out of three men with a PSA greater than 4.0 ng/ml has carcinoma (**Table 7.8**). A review of these and other series demonstrates the minimal importance of transrectal ultrasonography if there is an abnormality on DRE or elevated PSA. This has led to the widespread practice of performing TRUS only in men with either a palpable prostatic abnormality or an elevation in serum PSA or both.

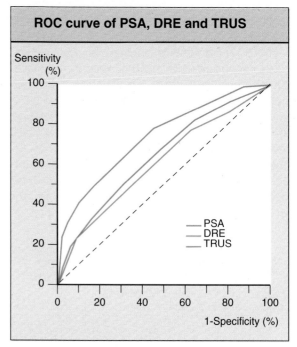

7.1 Receiver operating characteristic (ROC) curve comparing PSA, DRE and TRUS in a biopsy population. Note that overall PSA is the best predictor of carcinoma. (Reprinted from Ellis WJ, Chetner M, Preston S, *et al.* Diagnosis of prostatic carcinoma: the yield of serum PSA, DRE and TRUS. *J Urol* 1994;**152(5)**:1520–1525.)

Table 7.8 Yield of DRE, TRUS and PSA

DRE	TRUS	PSA	Catalona[35] BX/CaP (% CaP)	Cooner[32] BX/CaP (% CaP)	Lee[33] BX/CaP (% CaP)	Mettlin[61] BX/CaP (% CaP)	Brawer[72] BX/CaP (% CaP)	Total BX/CaP (% CaP)
–	–	–	11/0 (0)				23/0 (0)	37/0 (0)
–	–	+	37/6 (16)				53/10 (19)	90/26 (29)
+	–	–	17/0 (0)			30/5 (17)	78/5 (6)	125/10(8)
–	+	–	35/2 (6)	204/19 (9)	44/2 (5)	164/9 (6)	55/4 (7)	502/36 (7)
–	+	+	63/14 (22)	161/41 (25)	92/31 (34)	37/9 (24)	96/26 (27)	449/121 (27)
+	–	+	49/16 (33)			8/3 (38)	50/8 (16)	107/27 (25)
+	+	–	53/11 (21)	195/33 (17)	23/6 (26)	48/7 (15)	305/44 (14)	624/101 (16)
+	+	+	81/49 (60)	275/170 (62)	89/63 (71)	25/17 (68)	352/157 (45)	822/456 (56)

In an effort to improve the specificity for detection of prostate cancer, the concept of PSA index (PSAI, also referred to as PSA density) has emerged. Stamey and colleagues first reported that, volume for volume, prostatic carcinoma contributes ten times more to the serum PSA than benign prostatic hyperplasia[41].

Several authors have reported improvement in the predictive value of the calculated PSAI (that is, the PSA value divided by the calculated prostate volume in cm^3) as compared to serum PSA alone[42-44]. Benson evaluated 61 men with prostatic disease (41 with carcinoma undergoing radical prostatectomy and 20 with benign prostatic hyperplasia)[45]. The mean PSA density for prostate cancer was significantly greater than that for BPH. In a subsequent report, Benson and associates[46] evaluated 595 patients undergoing DRE and TRUS who were referred to a urological practice and were found to have PSA values between 4.1 and 10.0 ng/ml. Employing Student's t test, no significant difference was noted between the PSA levels in the patients undergoing biopsy who had positive and negative results. In contrast, PSA density calculations on those with and those without carcinoma were strongly significant.

In an attempt to confirm this observation, we compared serum PSA alone to PSA density in 218 men undergoing systematic, random, prostatic needle biopsy[47]. For the patient population as a whole, all methods of testing were approximately equivalent in their ability to provide a statistically significant ($p<0.01$) stratification between those patients with benign and malignant biopsies.

There may be several reasons for our inability to duplicate the results of Benson et al.[46]. The only way to resolve these differences between studies is to enroll patients in a prospective trial to evaluate the efficacy of PSA density in prostate cancer diagnosis. Such a study is currently being planned.

One interesting group presenting symptomatically comprises those men complaining of prostatic bladder-outlet obstruction. Incidental carcinoma of the prostate is found in 10–20% of men undergoing transurethral prostatectomy (TURP) for presumed benign disease[48]. In the American College of Surgeons review, nearly one half of all prostate cancer was found incidentally[49]. With the increasing utility of non-surgical or lesser-surgical approaches to the treatment of BPH, such as alpha adrenergic blockade, 5-alpha reductase inhibitors, laser prostatectomy, high-intensity focused ultrasound, hyperthermia, and so on, there is a genuine need for methods to discriminate between those patients with potentially clinically significant carcinoma and those with BPH alone.

We have evaluated 91 men seeking treatment in Seattle for bladder outlet obstruction with transrectal ultrasound (TRUS) and biopsy[50] (**Table 7.9**). The overall cancer-detection rate in this group was greater than that found in screening studies of asymptomatic men (13.2%). All cancers were found in men with either an abnormality on the DRE (including asymmetry), or a PSA greater than 4.0 ng/ml. Lepor has recently reported similar data[51].

SUMMARY OF SCREENING TESTS

Improvements in our diagnostic armamentarium have increased the sensitivity for subtle abnormalities on rectal examination, TRUS ultrasound-guided biopsy and most importantly PSA, and have truly revolutionized the detection of prostatic carcinoma. Several observations emerge from the numerous reports on the application of these to screening and early detection. As a single diagnostic test, PSA offers the best performance characteristics. Utilizing PSA, significantly higher positive predictive values are realized than that reported for mammography[52,53]. Even greater efficacy

Table 7.9 Histology of men with bladder-outlet obstruction undergoing TRUS biopsy

DRE	PSA (ng/ml)	Biopsy	CaP	% CaP
Normal	<4.0	47	0	0
	4.0–10.0	8	1	12.5
	>10.0	1	1	100.0
Asymmetry	<4.0	3	0	0
	4.0–10.0	0	0	0
	>10.0	0	0	0
Induration	<4.0	10	2	20.0
	4.1–10.0	8	2	25.0
	>10.0	6	3	50.0
'Malignant'	<4.0	5	1	20.0
	4.1–10.0	3	2	66.7
	>10.0	0	0	0
Total		91	12	

(positive predictive value) is realized if PSA is combined with DRE. PSA index, while intuitively making sense, seems in at least some settings to offer little more stratification of men who do or do not harbour malignancy than PSA alone. Transrectal ultrasound, while invaluable for performing biopsy, seems to add little to DRE and PSA in selecting men for biopsy.

Moreover, patients whose carcinomas are detected utilizing these modalities tend to have more favourable stage. For example, in Catalona et al.[35] as well as Brawer's PSA-based series[36], virtually all men had clinically localized malignancies (**Table 7.10**). While significant pathological upstaging was noted in the first year, with serial monitoring of the cohort, the vast majority of patients have organ-confined disease (**Table 7.11**).

PROBLEMS WITH SCREENING

Despite these encouraging observations, screening for prostate cancer may potentially give rise to significant problems (**Table 7.12**). Briefly, these may be divided into scientific, ethical, legal, and economic. In each of these domains, unfortunately, more questions remain about the efficacy of screening for prostate cancer than we have answers.

Problems in the scientific issues of screening include 'lead-' and 'length-time' bias as well as the very real potential of overdetection. Length-time bias has already been discussed. Lead-time bias occurs because, if we do nothing to alter the natural history with therapy, patients whose cancers are diagnosed as part of a

---

Table 7.10 Clinical stage in PSA screening patients

Clinical stage	Catalona et al.[35] (Year 1)	Brawer et al.[36] (Year 2)	Brawer et al.[37] (Year 3)	Brawer et al.[39]
		PSA > 4.0 ng/ml (%)		
NP	–	4 (33.3)	1 (14.3)	
B	–	8 (67.8)	6 (85.7)	
C	–	–	–	
D	–	–	–	
		PSA 4.0–10.0 ng/ml (%)		
NP	19 (100)	6 (26.1)	1 (50.0)	2 (40.0)
B	–	16 (69.6)	1 (50.0)	3 (60.0)
C	–	1 (4.3)	–	–
D	–	–	–	–
		PSA < 10.0 ng/ml (%)		
NP	10 (58.8)	2 (22.2)	1 (50.0)	1 (100.0)
B	–	6 (67.3)	1 (50.0)	–
C	7 (41.2)	1 (11.1)	–	–
D	–	–	–	–

–	Not specified
NP	Non-palpable
B	Confined neoplasm
C	Capsule penetrated or seminal vesicle invasion
D	Bony metastases

Table 7.11 Pathological stage in PSA screening patients

Pathological stage	Catalona et al.[35]	Brawer et al.[36] (Year 1)	Brawer et al.[37] (Year 2)	Brawer et al. (Year 3)
		PSA less than 4.0 ng/ml		
Organ confined, C1, C2, C3 and D1	–		6/8 (75/0)	2 (66.7)
	–	–	–	–
		PSA 4.0 to 10.0 ng/ml		
Organ confined, C1, C2, C3 and D1	10/17 (58.8)	9/12 (75.0)	1/8 (12.5)	1 (33.3)
	7/17 (41.2)	3/12 (25.0)	1/8 (12.5)	–
		PSA more than 10.0 ng/ml		
Organ confined, C1, C2, C3 and D1	2/16 (12.5)	–	–	
	14/16 (87.5)	4/4 (100.0)	–	–

Stage C1 = capsular penetration without perforation, Stage C2 = positive margin, Stage C3 = seminal-vesicle extension, and Stage D1 = pelvic lymph-node metastases.

screening programme will have a survival advantage (the lead time). However, no actual increased longevity may in fact be realized.

Overdetection is a significant issue in screening for prostatic carcinoma, perhaps more so than for any other malignancy. The discrepancy between prevalence and clinically manifest disease and the implications of this in screening have already been discussed.

Additional support for the potential lack of utility of early detection comes from the reports indicating the long natural history and the low cancer-related death rate owing to prostatic carcinoma in series of untreated patients previously described. It must be reiterated, however, that these derive from highly selected populations. Patient-selection bias, concurrent disease, tumour characteristics, and so on, make clear conclusions from these series difficult.

It seems obvious that some older men in whom cancer of the prostate is discovered may be better off untreated; however, one must balance this observation with the fact that all of the 3% of men destined to die of prostatic carcinoma at one point surely had curable neoplasms.

Many ethical dilemmas surround screening for prostate cancer. Society must decide the appropriate level of health resources to be applied to this disease. Certainly, the administration in Washington is scrutinizing the current approach in the US. Legal issues primarily surround the concept of informed consent.

Table 7.12 Prostate carcinoma screening: what we need to know

- Does treatment for localized prostate cancer result in a reduction in morbidity and mortality?

- Do screening tests identify patients who are curable and who need to be cured?

- What are the best screening tests to use, in whom and how often?

- Can we afford it?

Should a man undergo explanation of not only the potential benefits to be derived by application of screening tests but also the potential costs in terms of discomfort, morbidity, anxiety, as well as fiscal?

One of the biggest problems associated with prostate cancer screening is the tremendous potential cost incurred. The actual economic implications become increasingly significant when one realizes that the cost of early detection and screening is not merely the cost of the diagnostic test, even when it includes biopsy, pathology, staging and so forth. The true cost includes such factors as patient education, advertising for screening, treatment of complications of the diagnostic tests staging, definitive therapy, secondary therapy, monitoring of patients, and treatment of complications. Although several authors have estimated the cost likely to be incurred by widespread screening programmes based on various modelling approaches, the lack of unanimity of their conclusions mandates actual cost analysis of ongoing trials.

Several critical issues need to be answered before widespread recommendation of prostate cancer screening can be made (**Table 7.13**). We need prospective studies to definitively answer whether treatment for prostate cancer results in a decrease in mortality. This demands randomization of men into treatment and no-treatment arms with long follow-up, with both all-cause and cancer-related mortality being ascertained. Several studies are underway or have been planned. The Swedish Oncology Group is randomizing men to radical prostatectomy versus watchful waiting. In Denmark, men are being randomized to extended-beam radiation or expectant management. These studies are well-designed in that they offer randomization, but are unfortunately limited in the number of patients to be evaluated. Moreover, their Scandinavian setting may instill biases as we try to extrapolate the result of these investigations to populations in the rest of the world.

Recently initiated is the 'Prostatectomy Versus Observation for Clinically Localized Carcinoma of the Prostate' (PIVOT) trial, which will randomize 2000 men in the United States to radical prostatectomy versus expectant management. This trial, under the auspices of the Veterans Affairs Cooperative Study Program and the National Cancer Institute, is powered to detect a decrease in cancer-related mortality of 15%, and an overall decrease in mortality of 45%, and should defin-

itively answer the question of whether radical prostatectomy works in men with clinically localized disease[73]. Unfortunately, the results of the trial will not be known for many years; moreover, there are worries about the problems of recruiting into a study with a no-treatment arm.

Whether screening results in decreased cancer-related mortality remains to be proven. Obviously, as noted, this presupposes effective therapy, which should be answered by the above-mentioned studies. The PLCO trial (Prostate, Lung, Colon, Ovarian), funded by the National Cancer Institute and currently underway, randomizes men to screening with PSA and DRE versus no screening[74]. This large, cohort, multi-institutional trial utilizes cancer mortality as an end-point, and is an attempt to answer the question of whether early detection works. Unfortunately, no standard therapeutic regimens are provided, potentially resulting in significant biases. The biggest problem associated with this trial is whether indeed a non-screen population can still be identified in the USA where PSA testing is already prevalent. A pan-European screening project is also being organized which will have fewer problems in this respect.

In conclusion, screening for prostatic carcinoma is associated with the potential for both considerable problems and substantial benefits. How should the individual clinician proceed today? It seems appropriate that the gatekeeper – the individual who should make the decision whether or not early detection is warranted – should not be the urologist, but, more appropriately, that this decision should fall on the primary-care practitioner. He or she can weigh all of the evidence and factors surrounding the costs and benefits to accrue to the individual man. Factors to consider include the patient's overall health and intercurrent disease, socioeconomic considerations as well as physiological and chronological age and life expectancy. Only after appropriate and detailed counselling of the patient with regard to both the benefits and the potential risk of early detection of prostatic carcinoma can an appropriate decision be made.

If it is determined that it is in the best interests of the patient to be evaluated for prostatic cancer, then a carefully performed digital rectal examination and serum PSA determination should be accomplished. Biopsy should be performed for abnormality in either, ideally under sonographic guidance. The appropriate interval for such testing remains to be defined, but is probably about one year.

Table 7.13 Problems with screening
• Overdetection
• Unknown natural history
• Therapy unproven
• Economic
• Ethical
• Legal

If, after an analysis by the primary-care practitioner, it is not in the best interests of the patient to have an early diagnosis of prostatic carcinoma, because, for example, comorbidity suggests a life expectancy of < 10 years, then we believe no testing should be performed.

REFERENCES

1. American Cancer Society. Guidelines for the cancer-related health checkup: Recommendations and rationale. CA. 1980;**30**:194.
2. Boring CC, Squires TS, Tong T. Cancer statistics. CA Can J Clin. 1993;**43**:7–26.
3. Seidman H, Mushinski MH, Geib SK et al. Probabilities of eventually developing or dying of cancer – United States, 1985. CA. 1985;**35**:36–56.
4. Carter HB, Coffey D. The Prostate: An increasing medical problem. Prostate. 1990;**16(1)**;39–48.
5. Crawford ED. A controlled trial of leuprolide with and without flutamide in prostatic carcinoma. N Eng J Med. 1989;**321**:419–424.
6. Scardino PT, Gervasi L, Mata LA. The prognostic significance of the extent of nodal metastasis in prostatic cancer. J Urol. 1989;**142**:332–336.
7. Austenfield MS, Davis BE. New concepts in the treatment of stage D1 adenocarcinoma of the prostate. Urol Clin North America. 1990;**17**:867–884.
8. Zincke H, Utz D, Thule Pi, et al. Treatment options for patients with stage DI (TO–3, N1–2, Mo) adenocarcinoma of the prostate. Urology. 1987;**30**:307–315.
9. Smith J Jr, Haynes T, Middleton R. Impact of external irradiation on local symptoms and survival free of disease in pateints with pelvic lymph node metastasis from adenocarcinoma of the prostate. J Urol. 1984;**131**:705–707.
10. Mench HR, Garfinkel L, Dodd GD. Preliminary report of the National Cancer Data Base. CA. 1991;**41**:7–18.
11. Carlton CEJ, Scardino PT. (1988) Long-term results after combined radioactive gold seed implantation and external beam radiotherapy for localized prostatic cancer. In: A Multidisciplinary Analysis of Controversies in the Management of Prostate Cancer. Coffey, Resnick, Dorr (ed.) Plenum. New York.
12. Bagshaw MA. (1988) Radiation therapy for cancer of the prostate In: Diagnosis and Management of Genitourinary Cancer. Skinner, Lieskovsky (ed.) Saunders. Philadelphia.
13. Lepor H, Kimball AW, Walsh PC. Cause-specific actuarial survival analysis: A useful method for reporting survival data in men with clinically localized prostatic cancer: Long term results. J Urol. 1989;**141**:82–84.
14. Gibbons R, Correa R Jr, Brannen G, et al. Total prostatectomy for clinically localized prostatic cancer: Long–term results. J Urol 1989;**131**:564–566.
15. Paulson DF, Moul JW, Walter PJ. Radical prostatectomy for stage T1–2 NO MO prostatic adenocarcinoma, long term results. J Urol 1990;**144**(5):1180–1184.
16. McNeal JE, Bostwick DG, Kindrachuck RA, et al. Patterns of progression in prostate cancer. Lancet. 1986;**1**:60–63.
17. Franks LM. Latency and progression in tumors: The natural history of prostatic cancer. Lancet. 1956;**2**:1037.
18. Dhom G. Epidemiologic aspects of latent and clinically manifest carcinoma of the prostate. J Cancer Res Clin Oncol. 1983;**106**:210.
19. Scott R Jr, Mutchnik DL, Laskowski TZ et al. Carcinoma of the prostate in elderly men: Incidence, growth characteristics and clinical significance. J Urol. 1969;**101**:602–607.
20. Kabalin JN, McNeal JE, Price HM, et al. Unsuspected adenocarcinoma of the prostate in patients undergoing cystoprostatectomy for other causes: Incidence, histology and morphometric observations. J Urol. 1989;**141**:1091–1094.
21. Montie JE, Wood DP Jr, Pontes JE, et al. Adenocarcinoma of the prostate in cystoprostatectomy specimens removed for bladder cancer. Cancer 1989;**63**:381–385.
22. Babaian RJ, Troncoso P, Ayala A. Transurethral resection zone prostate cancer detected at cystoprostatectomy. Cancer 1991;**67**:1418–1422.
23. Troncoso P, Babaian RJ, Ro JY, et al. Prostatic intraepithelial neoplasia and invasive prostatic adenocarcinoma in cysto-prostatectomy specimens. Urology 1989;**34**(Suppl):52–56.
24. Scardino PT. Early detection of prostate cancer. Urol Clin North Am. 1989;**16**:635–655.
25. Johansson J-E, Adami H, Andersson S-O, et al. High 10-year survival rate in patients with early, untreated prostatic cancer. JAMA. 1992;**267**:2191–2196.
26. Whitmore W Jr, Warner J, Thompson I Jr. Expectant management of localized prostatic cancer. Cancer. 1991;**67**:1091–1096.
27. Hanash K, Cooke E, Taylor W, et al. Carcinoma of the prostate: A 15-year follow-up. J Urol. 1972;**107**: 450–453.
28. George NJR. Natural history of localized prostatic cancer managed by conservative therapy alone. Lancet 1988;**110**: 95–100.
29. Madsen PO, Graverson PH, Gasser TC, et al. Treatment of localized prostatic cancer: Radical prostectomy vs. placebo: A 15-year followup. Scand J Urol Nephrol Suppl. 1988;**110**:95–100.
30. Johansson JE, Adami HO, Andersson SO, et al. Natural history of localized prostatic cancer. A population-based study in 223 untreated patients. Lancet 1989;**1**:799–803.
31. Scardino PT, Weaver R, Hudson MA. Early detection of prostate cancer. Human Pathology 1992;**23**(3):211–222.
32. Cooner W, Mosley R, Rutherford CJ, et al. Prostate cancer detection in a clinical urological practice by ultrasonography, digital rectal examination and prostate specific antigen. J. Urol. 1990;**143**:1146–1152.
33. Lee F, Littrup PJ, Torp-Pederson ST, et al. Prostate cancer: Comparison of transrectal US and DRE for screening. Radiology 1988;**168**: 389–394.
34. Drago JR. The role of new modalities in the early detection and diagnosis of prostate cancer. CA. 1990;**40**:77.
35. Catalona W, Smith D, Ratcliff T, et al. Measurement of prostate-specific antigen in serum as a screening test for prostate cancer. N. Engl. J Med. 1991;**324**:1156–1161.
36. Brawer M, Chetner M, Beatie J, et al. Screening for prostatic carcinoma with prostate-specific antigen. J. Urol. 1992;**147**: 841–845.

37. Kirby RS, Kirby MG, Feneley MR, *et al*. Screening for prostate cancer: a GP based study. Br J Urol 1994;**74**:64–71.

38. Chadwick DJ, Kemple T, Astley JP, *et al*. Pilot study of screening for prostate cancer in general practice. *Lancet* 1991;**338**:613–616.

39 Brawer MK, Beattie J, Wener MH, *et al*. Screening for prostatic carcinoma with prostate specific antigen: Results of the second year. J. Urol. 1993;**150**:106–109.

40. Schmid HP, McNeal JE, Stamey TA. Observations on the doubling time of prostate cancer: The use of serial prostate specific antigen in patients with untreated disease as a measure of increasing cancer volume. CA. 1993;**71**(6):2031.

41. Stamey T, Yang N, Hay AR, *et al*. Prostate-specific antigen as a serum marker for adenocarcinoma of the prostate. N *Engl J Med*. 1987;**317**:909–916.

42. Habib GK, Bissas A, Neill WA, *et al*. Flow cytometric analysis of cellular DNA in human prostate cancer: relationship to 5-alpha reductase activity of the tissue. Urol Res. 1989;**17**:239.

43. Fair WR, Presti JC, Sogani B, *et al*. Multicenter, randomized, double-blind, placebo controlled study to investigate the effect of finasteride (MK-906) on stage D prostate cancer. J Urol. 1991;**145**:317A.

44. Gormley GJ, Stoner E, Bruskewitz RC, *et al*. The effect of finasteride in men with benign prostatic hyperplasia. N *Engl J Med*. 1992;**327**:1185.

45. Benson M, Whang I, Pantuck A, *et al*. Prostate specific antigen density: A means of distinguishing benign prostatic hypertrophy and prostate cancer. J Urol. 1992;**147**:815–816.

46. Benson M, Whang I, Olsson C, *et al*.. The use of prostate-specific antigen density to enhance the predictive value of intermediate levels of serum prostate–specific antigen. J. Urol. 1992;**147**:817–821.

47. Brawer MK, Aramburu EAG, Chen GL, *et al*. The inability of prostate specific antigen index to enhance the predictive value of prostate specific antigen in the diagnosis of prostatic carcinoma. J Urol. 1993;**150**:369.

48. Altwein JE, Faul P, Schneider W. *Incidental Carcinoma of the Prostate*. 1991, Springer-Verlag, Berlin.

49. Schmidt JD, Mettlin CJ, Natarajan N, *et al*. Trends in patterns of care for prostatic cancer, 1974–1983: Results of surveys by the American College of Surgeons. J. Urol. 1986;**136**:416–421.

50. Ploch NR, Ellis WJ, Brawer MK. Transrectal ultrasound guided prostate needle biopsies in men presenting with obstructive voiding symptoms. 1994 AUA Annual Meeting. 1993.

51. Lepor H, Owens RS, Rogenes V, *et al*. Detection of prostate cancer in men with prostatism. *Prostate* 1994;**25**:132–148.

52. Kinne DW, Kopans DB. Physical examination and mammography in the diagnosis of breast disease. *Breast Disease*. 1987:54–86.

53. Moskowitz M. Cost-benefit determinations in screening mammography. CA *Suppl*. 1987;**60**:1680–1683.

54. Catalona WJ, Smith DS, Ratliff TL. Value of measurements of the rate of change on serum PSA levels in prostate cancer screening. J Urol. 1993;**149**(4): 300A.

55. Chodak GW, Schoenberg HW. Progress and problems in screening for carcinoma of the prostate. *World J Surg*. 1989;**13**:60–64.

56. Faul P. Experience with the German annual preventive checkup examination. In: *Prostate Cancer*. 1982;57.

57. Gilbertsen VA. Cancer of the prostate gland: Results of early diagnosis and therapy undertaken for cure of the disease. JAMA. 1976;**215**: 81–84.

58. Jenson CB, Shahon DB, Wangensteen OH. Evaluation of annual examinations in the detection of cancer: Special reference to cancer of the gastrointestinal tract, prostate, breast, and female reproductive tract. JAMA. 1960;**174**: 1783–1788.

59. Lee F, Littrup P, Torp-Pedersen S, *et al*. Prostate cancer: Comparison of transrectal US and digital rectal examination for screening. *Radiology* 1988;**168**:389–394.

60. McWhorter WP, Hernandez AD, Meikle AW, *et al*. A screening study prostate cancer in high risk families. J Urol. 1992;**148**: 826.

61. Mettlin C, Lee F, Drago J, *et al*.. The American Cancer Society National Prostate Cancer Detection Project: Findings on the detection of early prostate cancer in 2425 men. *Cancer*. 1991;**67**:2949–2958.

62. Mueller EJ, Crain TW, Thompson IM, *et al*. An evaluation of serial digital rectal examinations in screening for prostate cancer. J Urol. 1988;**140**:1445.

63. Thompson IM, Rounder JB, Teaque JL, *et al*. Impact of routine screening for adenocarcinoma of the prostate on stage distribution. J Urol. 1987;**137**:424.

64. Vihko P, Kontturi M, Lukkarinen O, *et al*. Screening for carcinoma of the prostate: Rectal examination, and enzymatic and radioimmunologic measurements of serum acid phosphatase compared. *Cancer*. 1985;**56**:173–177.

65. Waaler G, Ludvigsen TC, Runden TO, *et al*. Digital rectal examination to screen for prostatic cancer. *Eur Urol*. 1988;**15**:34.

66. Devonec M, Chapeleon JY, Cathignol D. Comparison of the diagnostic value of sonography and rectal examination in cancer of the prostate. *Eur Urol*. 1988;**14**:189.

67. Fritzche PJ, Axford PO, Ching VC, *et al*. Correlation of transrectal sonographic findings in patients with suspected and unsuspected prostatic disease. J Urol. 1983;**30**:272.

68. Hunter PT, Butler SA, Hodge GB, *et al*. Detection of prostatic cancer using transrectal ultrasound and sonographically guided biopsy in 1410 symptomatic. J Endourol. 1989;**3**:167.

69. Perrin P, Mouriquand P, Monsallier M, *et al*. Irradiation of carcinoma of the prostate localized to the pelvis: Analysis of tumor response and prognosis. Int J *Radiat Oncol Biol Phys*. 1980;**6**:555.

70. Ragde H, Bagley CM, Aldpae HC, *et al*. Screening for prostatic cancer with high–resolution ultrasound. J Endourol. 1989;**3**:115.

71. Rifkin MD, Friedland GW, Shortliffe L. Prostatic evaluation by transrectal ultrasonography: Detection of carcinoma. *Radiology* 1986;**158**:85.

72. Brawer MK. Unpublished Observation.

73. Wilt TJ, Brawer MK. Prostate cancer intervention versus observation trial: randomized trial comparing radical prostatectomy versus expectant management for the treatment of clinically localized cancer. J Urol 1994;**152**:1910–1921.

74. Gohagan JK, Prorok PC, Kramer BS, *et al*. Prostate cancer screening in prostate, lung, colorectal and ovarian cancer screening trial of National Cancer Institute. J Urol 1994;**152**:1905–1909.

CHAPTER 8

IMAGING AND STAGING OF PROSTATE CANCER

INTRODUCTION

As mentioned in Chapter 5, a patient's clinical history and physical examination, in isolation, are not always reliable in guiding the clinician towards a diagnosis of prostate cancer. With the additional assistance of various imaging modalities, the urologist will, in the majority of cases, be able to confirm the diagnosis of clinically significant prostate cancer by ultrasound guided biopsies, and to provide a reasonable but imperfect estimate of the stage of the cancer. Digital

rectal examination (DRE) is only 30–50% accurate in the diagnosis of prostate cancer, and often underestimates[1], but sometimes overestimates, the local extent of the disease[2]. Therefore, the steady improvements in imaging to permit more accurate staging represent a significant advance. More accurate staging, and particularly the differentiation between confined prostate cancer and extra-capsular spread and seminal-vesicle involvement, is vital for the selection of those patients who would derive a long-term survival benefit from interventions such as radical prostatectomy.

IMAGING FOR LOCALIZED PROSTATE CANCER

Intravenous Urography

In locally advanced cases, prostate cancer may present initially with symptoms of bladder-outflow obstruction. Although ultrasonography is the usual imaging technique of choice in such circumstances, some urologists still request intravenous urography in men with bladder-outflow symptoms. Prostate cancer may also present with haematuria (macroscopic or microscopic) and/or loin pain, which are the main indications for excretory urography. The possible findings in intravenous urography in prostate cancer are outlined in **Table 8.1** and can be divided broadly into bony, renal, ureteric and bladder abnormalities.Intravenous urography should not be considered as a necessary investigation in the diagnosis or investigation of prostate cancer, but may reveal abnormalities that warrant further investigation to confirm the presence of underlying prostate cancer (**8.1**).

Transabdominal Ultrasound

Imaging of the prostate by ultrasonography was originally performed transabdominally, but the interpretation of the images is sometimes difficult due to interfaces between other intra-abdominal structures. However, ultrasonic examination of the bladder and

Table 8.1 Intravenous urography in prostate cancer: possible findings

Skeleton	Bony metastases - osteosclerotic (98%) - osteolytic (2%) Osteomalacia secondary to renal failure or secondary hyperparathyroidism
Kidneys	Hydronephrosis (one or both kidneys) Non-functioning kidney (usually one)
Ureters	Obstruction due to extrinsic compression by lymph node metastases Distal obstruction from local extension
Bladder	Calculi within bladder Trabeculation Diverticula Prostatic impression at bladder base Post-micturition residual

the measurement of the pre-micturition and post-micturition volumes are important investigations in the assessment of outflow obstruction caused by the prostate, and encroachment of the median prostate into the bladder may be well visualized by this means (**8.2**). Transabdominal-ultrasound scanning is best combined with uroflowmetry to give an estimation of the severity of bladder-outflow obstruction (**8.3**).

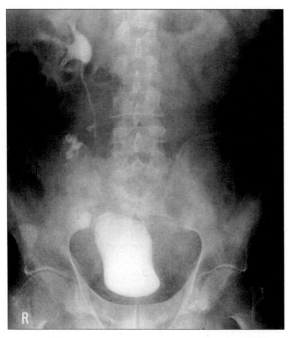

8.1 An IVU showing distortion of the bladder by pelvic lymph nodes enlarged by prostate cancer and a non-functioning left kidney.

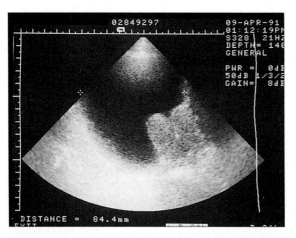

8.2 Encroachment of the bladder by prostatic tissue as visualized on transabdominal ultrasound.

Transrectal Ultrasound (TRUS)

Although more uncomfortable and intrusive than transabdominal scanning, transrectal ultrasound (TRUS) scanning has the distinct advantage of greater acuity resulting from the very close approximation of the probe to the prostate (**Table 8.2**). Technological advances in ultrasound equipment, particularly B-mode, grey-scale imaging, high frequency transducers (7–7.5 MHz) and colour Doppler, have enabled significant improvements in the accuracy of scanning of the prostate.

Equipment

TRUS is performed with an endorectal probe which is usually hand-held. Some of the early devices incorporated the probe in a chair, but these are now outmoded since they do not permit accurate movement of the probe to scan the entire prostate, and do not allow the operator to perform biopsies with ease. The endorectal probes come in all sorts of shapes and sizes and are very similar to the endovaginal probes used by gynaecologists. If an air interface becomes interposed between the probe and the prostate the image will deteriorate, and for this reason some probes incorporate a surrounding condom filled with degassed water. A number of technical improvements are usual in contemporary probes. Most probes have

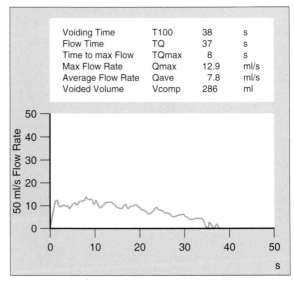

8.3 A uroflow recording from a patient with both BPH and localized prostate cancer suggesting obstruction.

7.5 MHz transducers which provide a spatial resolution down to 0.2 mm. Biplanar scanning in the sagittal and transverse axial planes enables more complete scanning of the prostate. Another technical refinement is colour Doppler; this enhancement enables the assessment of blood flow within regions of the prostate which may help with diagnosis, particularly in regard to distinguishing between malignancy and inflammation (i.e. prostatitis).

Technique
Prior to scanning, it is important to ensure that the rectum is clear of stool, since interposition of faecal material between the probe and the anterior rectal wall will distort the image. (This may be achieved by the use of an enema.) The patient is usually positioned in the left lateral, knee-to-chest position (**8.4**), although some prefer to scan with the patient in the dorsal lithotomy position. The tip of the probe should be well

lubricated prior to insertion. It is usual practice to initially scan the prostate in the transverse axial plane in a step-wise fashion from the base of the bladder down to the apex of the prostate. Glandular asymmetry and abnormalities within the prostate and seminal vesicles may become apparent. Next, step-wise scanning is performed in the longitudinal plane to identify any abnormalities not apparent on transverse scanning, and to estimate the three-dimensional characteristics of abnormalities apparent on transverse scanning.

Most scanners now incorporate a measuring cursor that can be used to estimate the total prostate volume and the volume of tumours within the prostate. The volume of the prostate can be calculated using the prolate ellipse formula: volume = 0.52 × Length × Width × Height (axial)[3] (**Table 8.3**). Some TRUS scanners also incorporate software capable of calculating prostate volume by drawing around the periphery of the prostate with a cursor on both longitudinal and transverse scans. Measurement of the prostate volume is a prerequisite for estimating the PSA density (PSAD) (see Chapter 7), and can also be used to determine the response in terms of reduction of prostate volume to various systemic and local therapies.

TRUS findings
Normal Prostate
On TRUS, the normal prostate has sharply defined, symmetrical contours and is homogeneous (**Table 8.4**). The prostate is surrounded by a discrete smooth 'capsule' which is hypoechoic due to the presence of periprostatic fat. The seminal vesicles, which are readily identifiable, are hypoechoic, symmetrical and sacculated.

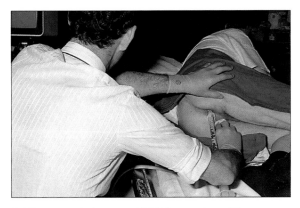

8.4 Transrectal ultrasound (TRUS) scanning of the prostate is usually performed with the patient in the left lateral position.

Table 8.2 Objectives of TRUS imaging in prostate cancer
Prostate volume measurement
Early diagnosis
Biopsy guidance
Staging
Detection of post-treatment recurrence

Table 8.3 Calculation of prostate volume by TRUS
Volume = 0.52 × (L × W × H)
L = Length on longitudinal scanning
W = Width on transverse axial scanning
H = Height on transverse axial scanning

Benign Prostatic Hyperplasia

In early BPH, the anteroposterior diameter of the prostate increases due to a relatively homogeneous enlargement of the transition zone. With enlargement of the transition zone in BPH, the peripheral zone may become compressed and hyperechoic, leading to a clear, ultrasonographic margin between the two zones (**8.5**). Discrete nodules of BPH or 'adenomas', which may be hypoechoic or less commonly hyperechoic, can distort the external contours of the prostate, and are often visualized within the transition zone; they may be difficult to differentiate from prostate cancer[4]. Large nodules of BPH are sometimes surrounded by a hypoechoic halo. Prostatic calculi are also a common feature in BPH, and are usually located at the junction between the posterolateral transition zone and the peripheral zone. Cystic degeneration may occur within BPH tissue and the hypoechoic appearance that this produces may be confused with cancer.

Table 8.4 Normal prostate zonal constitution on TRUS	
Peripheral zone	70%
Central zone	20%
Transition zone	10%

Prostatitis

In acute prostatitis, TRUS is often indistinguishable from BPH or indeed carcinoma. However, in chronic prostatitis there are a number of identifying features: an echo-free halo surrounding an echogenic area in the anterior periurethral area, hypoechoic areas within the parenchyma and anechoic linear structures surrounding the prostate. The increased vascularity that is associated with inflammation shows up well on colour Doppler imaging (**8.6**). There may also be abnormal prominence of periprostatic veins.

Prostate Cancer

Many (but by no means all) prostate cancers are hypoechoic on TRUS (**8.7a** and **8.7b**), but they may also be isoechoic and sometimes hyperechoic (**Table 8.5**). Prostate cancers most commonly develop within the peripheral zone, but can develop in the transition zone which is itself hypoechoic (**Table 8.6**). Even in the peripheral zone there are other causes for hypoechoic areas, and the specificity of this finding for prostate cancer is only 20–25%[4]. Other TRUS characteristics of prostate cancer include asymmetry of size, shape and echogenicity, indiscrete differentiation between the central and peripheral zones, and disruption of the capsule (**Table 8.7**).

TRUS is important in prostate cancer not only in making the diagnosis, but also in staging the disease. It is particularly relevant to determine if there is any evidence of extracapsular extension (ECE). Bulging, or irregularity of the boundary echo adjacent to a peripheral-zone hypoechoic lesion, is a relatively specific feature of capsular extension[5,6]. Invasion of the seminal vesicles may also be apparent on TRUS.

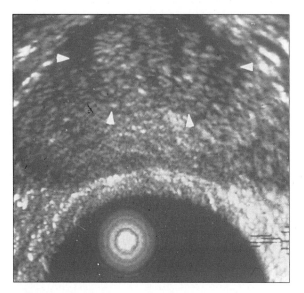

8.5 BPH on TRUS showing enlargement of the hypoechoic transition zone (arrowed).

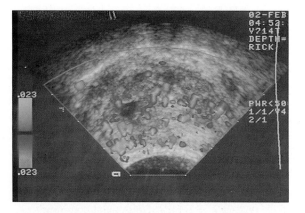

8.6 Colour Doppler TRUS demonstrating markedly increased blood flow characteristic of the inflammation resulting from acute prostatitis.

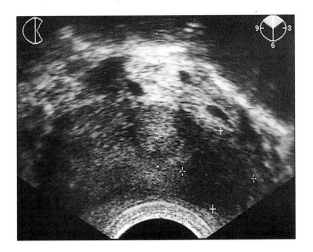

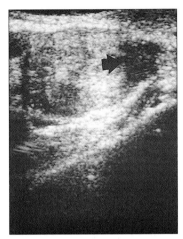

8.7 Hypoechoic lesion on TRUS: transverse plane (above); longitudinal imaging (left).

If extensive ECE is present, this would be considered by most to be a contraindication for radical prostatectomy. However, the detection of limited capsular involvement might help guide the surgeon in performing radical prostatectomy. A more extensive procedure, including excision of the neurovascular bundle adjacent to the ECE, might enable the urologist to achieve complete tumour removal. Although TRUS in isolation is reasonably accurate in determining the presence of ECE, it is now apparent that consideration of DRE findings in conjunction with TRUS can, in the best centres, achieve a reasonable specificity in the detection of capsular extension[6].

TRUS-guided biopsy

As in any other cancer, histological confirmation is an essential prerequisite before planning treatment for prostate cancer. A number of different biopsy techniques have been used. Digital guidance can be used to direct the biopsy of palpable lesions via the transrectal or transperineal routes. However, TRUS guidance has been shown to be superior to digital guidance in directing biopsy of both palpable and impalpable prostate cancers. Since TRUS is of additional benefit in staging prostate cancer, it makes practical sense to perform all prostate biopsies under TRUS guidance. There has been some discussion regarding the route for biopsy. The transperineal route carries the advantage that it is less likely to introduce infection, but the disadvantages of requiring local anaesthesia and being less easy to guide with the TRUS probe. In contrast, the transrectal route can be utilized without the need for injection of local anaesthesia, and can be guided accurately through the biopsy port incorporated in the TRUS probe. It is now standard practice to administer a broad-spectrum intravenous antibiotic prior to biopsy, and to give a three-day course of oral antibiotics after the biopsy. Controversy has surrounded the

Table 8.5 TRUS features of localized prostate cancer

Echogenicity	Percentage
Hypoechoic	68%
Isoechoic	31%
Hyperechoic	1%

Table 8.6 Site of origin of prostate cancer

Peripheral zone	70%
Transition zone	20%
Central zone	10%

Table 8.7 Characteristic features of prostate cancer on TRUS

Abnormal echo patterns

Loss of differentiation between central and peripheral zones

Asymmetry of size or shape

Distortion of the capsule

technique for the biopsy itself. Fine-needle aspiration has been advocated by some, but the cellular aspirate is sometimes difficult to interpret cytologically, resulting in a false negative diagnosis. A study comparing aspiration cytology with core biopsy in 30 patients with prostate cancer showed that whilst core biopsy made the correct diagnosis in all cases, there was a false positive rate of 30% for aspiration cytology[7]. Most prostatic biopsies are now accomplished using automatic biopsy devices (**8.8**, **8.9**).

Transurethral Ultrasound

Ultrasound probes that are small enough to be inserted transurethrally have also been developed and used to scan the prostate from within the prostatic urethra. The architecture of the prostate can be assessed and its volume measured using such probes[8]. However, general anaesthesia is usually necessary for insertion of the probe and the presence of the probe within the prostatic urethra can lead to distortion of the contours of the prostate. TRUS is considered to be superior to transurethral ultrasound as a scanning method for the prostate.

Computed Tomography

The advent of computerized tomography (CT) – the first technique to produce cross-sectional images – brought fresh hopes that it might be possible to accurately stage localized prostate cancer and to demonstrate metastases within pelvic lymph nodes. However, although the acuity of CT scanning can be great, interpretation of the scans has been disappointingly inaccurate in terms of local staging. The sensitivity of CT scanning in the detection of ECE and seminal-vesicle invasion has been reported as only 18–50%[9]. Furthermore, CT scanning also has a low specificity for ECE and seminal-vesicle invasion due to a high false positive rate. It is generally considered that CT scanning is less accurate than transabdominal ultrasound and TRUS in the local staging of prostate cancer[10].

Visualization of large-volume, lymph-node metastases is certainly possible with CT scanning (**8.10**), and the technique may also permit skinny-needle aspiration under CT control (**8.11**). However, lymph-node metastases, when present in prostate cancer, often do not produce conspicuous enlargement of the lymph glands and therefore may be undetectable by CT.

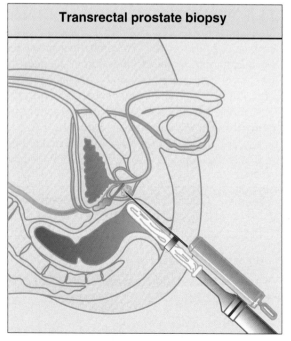

8.8 The technique of TRUS-guided automatic needle biopsy of the prostate.

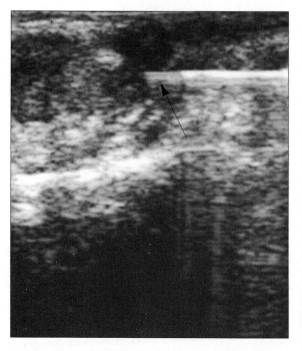

8.9 The TRUS-guided needle entering the prostate seen (arrowed) on ultrasound.

Magnetic Resonance Imaging

Magnetic resonance imaging (MRI) is a new and rapidly advancing, but expensive, technique that uses a magnetic field, rather than ionizing radiation, to produce images of startling clarity[11]. The patient is placed within a scanner which creates an intense uniform magnetic field that aligns the rotational axes of atomic nuclei, particularly protons. A short, powerful pulse of radiofrequency energy is then applied, leading to a change in the energy levels of the atomic nuclei. When the radiofrequency pulse stops, the nuclei return to their original energy level, and in doing so emit energy that can be received and transformed into an image pattern. This return to the previous equilibrium state after the energy pulse is called magnetic relaxation. Two relaxation time measurements can be used to produce varying images. The T1 relaxation time represents the regrowth of the longitudinal component, and the T2 relaxation time is the exponential time decay constant. Use of both T1 and T2 measurements can be used to produce complementary images. MRI scanners are capable of producing images in the tranverse axial, coronal and sagittal planes, and endorectal probes are now available for enhanced definition.

On T1-weighted images, it is not possible to demonstrate the internal architecture of the prostate, although a clear demarcation is apparent between the prostate and seminal vesicles and the surrounding fat. In contrast, T2-weighted MRI images are able to demonstrate clearly the internal architecture of the prostate (**8.12**). Typically, the peripheral zone of the prostate returns high intensity signals, whilst prostate cancer produces relatively low intensity signals. However, most other abnormalities within the prostate such as 'adenomas', corpora amylacea and prostatitis also return low intensity signals, so that MRI is unfortunately not especially accurate at identifying localized prostate cancer. Disappointingly, MRI has not proven very much more accurate than TRUS in local staging of prostate cancer, but the supplementation of tranverse axial scans with coronal and sagittal scanning has been shown to enhance local staging accuracy from 61–83%. Extracapsular extension is likely if there is apparent asymmetry, irregularity or breaching of the periprostatic fat which, unlike the prostate itself, sends low intensity signals (**8.13**, **8.14**). Seminal-vesicle invasion is suggested if there are areas of asymmetric low intensity within the normally high intensity vesicles[12].

A recent multicentre trial comparing MRI with TRUS in the staging of localized prostate cancer concluded that there was no statistically significant difference between the two[13]. However, it is generally accepted that TRUS is marginally more accurate than MRI in the differentiation of stage B and stage C prostate cancer,

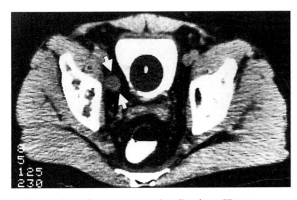

8.10 Lymph-node metastases visualized on CT scan (arrowed).

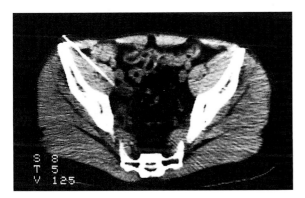

8.11 CT-guided skinny-needle aspiration of enlarged lymph node in a patient with prostate cancer.

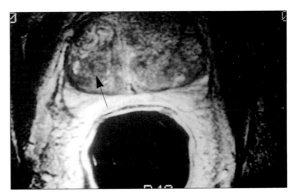

8.12 T2-weighted MRI of the prostate showing nodular areas of benign prostatic hyperplasia (arrowed).

and that TRUS should still be considered as the 'gold-standard' imaging modality for prostate malignancy.

There is undoubtedly the prospect of more accurate staging of localized prostate cancer. Ever-improving intracavity and MRI surface coils are currently being evaluated. The images of the internal architecture of the prostate produced from these devices are of exceedingly high quality[14]. It seems probable that endorectal MRI scanning will eventually prove to be more accurate than current techniques in the local staging of prostate malignancy, although cost constraints may always limit their availability for every patient.

IMAGING FOR METASTATIC PROSTATE CANCER

Lymphangiography

Pedal lymphangiography was once a popular technique for imaging pelvic lymph nodes. However, the technique is invasive, uncomfortable for the patient, time-consuming, and carries the risk of morbidity from pulmonary embolism due to the lipid-based contrast medium. With the advent of CT and MRI scanning the use of lymphangiography has virtually fallen into abeyance. Nevertheless, lymphangiography, by examining the internal architecture of lymph nodes, does provide images that cannot be duplicated by other techniques, although metastases must be at least 5 mm in diameter to be detectable. Good images can be obtained of the external iliac, common iliac and para-aortic nodes, but some doubt has been cast upon the ability of lymphangiography to adequately image the hypogastric and obturator nodes, which are precisely those which become involved earliest in the natural history of metastatic prostate cancer. The accuracy of lymphangiography has been tested in 40 patients who subsequently underwent open pelvic lymphadenectomy as a staging manoeuvre for prostate. Lymphangiography produced a false positive rate of 59% and a false negative rate of 36%[14]. Most urologists accept that lymphangiography now has little role to play in contemporary clinical practice in staging prostate cancer.

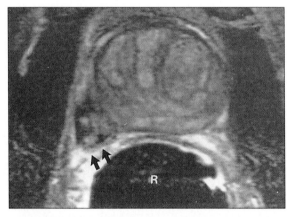

8.13 T2-weighted MRI of prostate showing cancer in peripheral zone infiltrating the neurovascular bundle on that side (arrowed); R = rectum.

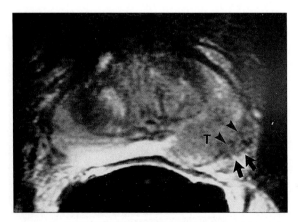

8.14 MRI showing extra capsular extension (ECE) by prostate cancer (arrowed).

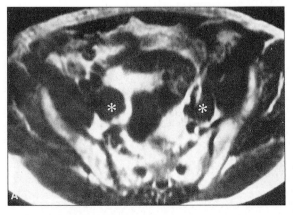

8.15 Lymph-node metastases from prostate cancer visualized on MRI (starred).

Computed Tomography

CT scanning is complementary to lymphangiography in the detection of lymph-node metastases in prostate cancer. However, CT scanning is only 40–50% accurate in identifying metastatic involvement of pelvic lymph nodes since it relies upon enlargement of the nodes

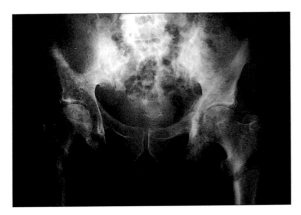

8.16 Osteosclerotic bony metastases in sacrum and pelvis from prostate cancer seen on plain x-ray.

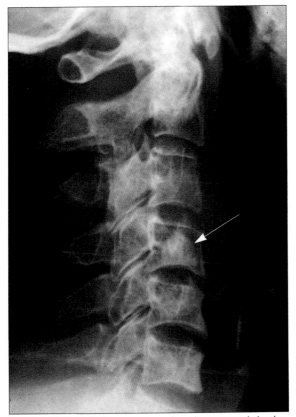

8.17(a) X-ray showing an osteosclerotic metastasis in the cervical spine (arrowed).

and will therefore miss small and microscopic metastases. Large, pelvic lymph-node metastases are more likely to be detected at pelvic CT scanning in men with a large primary tumour and in those with a PSA >20.

Magnetic Resonance Imaging

As with CT scanning, MRI scanning relies upon size criteria in the diagnosis of pelvic lymph-node metastases (**8.15**). It is therefore not surprising that the sensitivity of MRI in detecting lymph-node metastases is less than 10%, although the specificity is higher at over 90% since obvious nodal enlargement on scanning generally represents metastatic disease. There is no evidence to suggest that MRI is superior to CT scanning in the detection of nodal metastases from prostate cancer, and the technique is more expensive and demanding on the patient because of the claustrophobic nature of the scanner.

Plain Roentgenography

Plain roentgenography has little role to play in the routine diagnosis or investigation of prostate cancer. However, plain x-ray films taken in the course of performing intravenous urography in men with prostate cancer may reveal bony metastases, especially within the pelvic bones and lower lumbar spine (**8.16**). Bony metastases in prostate cancer are osteosclerotic (increase in bone density) in 98% of cases (**8.17a**), and osteolytic (decrease in bone density) in only 2%. The main indication for the use of plain roentgenography in prostate cancer is to further investigate areas of the body that reveal suspicious, but equivocally metastatic, areas on radioisotope bone scanning. Very occasionally, bone biopsies may be needed to confirm the diagnosis (**8.17b**).

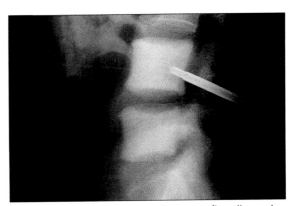

(b) Bone biopsy from lumbar spine to confirm diagnosis of metastatic prostate cancer under x-ray control.

Roentgenographic skeletal surveys in men with known prostate cancer are now rarely indicated and are anyway rather inaccurate. Before metastases become apparent within the skeleton on plain roentgenography, they have to reach about 1.5 cm in diameter and replace 50–70% of the bone, and there is often a delay period of 3–6 months before metastases visualized on radionucleotide bone scanning become obvious on plain roentgenography[15]. For these reasons, plain roentgenography in the form of skeletal survey has been largely superseded by radionucleotide scanning.

Radionuclide Bone Scanning

Radionuclide bone scanning has been extensively used since the 1960s, with the most popular isotope utilized being Technetium. Total body scanning examines the entire skeleton; the total scanning time is about one hour and is performed about three hours after injecting the isotope. It is usual practice to perform a bone scan at the time of initial diagnosis of prostate cancer (**8.18a** and **b**).

Although isotope bone scanning is more sensitive than plain roentgenography, serum acid phosphatase and serum alkaline phosphatase in the detection of bony metastases from prostate cancer, the use of bone scans in the routine follow-up of prostate cancer patients has fallen out of favour since the advent of PSA testing, as PSA has proven to be the best predictor of bone-scan positivity. A study of 521 men has revealed only one man with a positive bone scan and PSA less than 20 ng/ml. Therefore the negative predictive value for PSA <20 ng/ml is 99.7% (**Table 8.8**). It could be argued that the 50% or more of men with prostate cancer who now present with PSA <20 ng/ml may not require a bone scan[16]. Follow-up of prostate cancer patients with bony metastases is most accurately and cost-effectively done by measuring serum PSA rather than repeat radionuclide bone scans[17].

False positive results can occur in the presence of arthritis, old bone fractures, osteomyelitis, trauma and previous surgery. If any doubt exists about areas apparent on bone scans then a plain roentgenograph should be performed. In some cases, however, these will also not be diagnostic, and bone biopsy can be performed to confirm the diagnosis (**8.17a, b**). False negative bone scans may occur with small symmetrical lesions. An unusual but sometimes dramatic finding on bone scan is the so-called 'superscan' in which the whole skeleton appears to take up the radioisotope at high density.

Laparoscopic Pelvic Lymphadenectomy

Perhaps because lymph nodes involved by prostate cancer are often indurated but not markedly enlarged, non-invasive imaging has been rather disappointing as a means of accurate evaluation of the obturator and hypogastric lymph nodes. In the past, therefore, lymph-node staging has been performed by an open operation, either as a staging procedure prior to radiotherapy or radical perineal prostatectomy, or as part of radical retropubic prostatectomy. There now exists, however, the possibility of undertaking this procedure using minimally invasive techniques of laparoscopic technology. Laparoscopic pelvic lymphadenectomy (LPLND) is now a feasible option which allows accurate evaluation of the nodal status of patients with minimal attendant morbidity. The post-operative hospital stay is only 24–48 hours and most patients return to work within a week.

Clearly, pelvic lymph-node dissection is not appropriate for every patient, but should perhaps be considered in individuals with either higher Gleason score (>6) prostate cancer on biopsy, or a PSA greater than 20 ng/ml who have no other evidence of metastatic disease and who are candidates, by virtue of tumour stage and their life expectancy, for curative therapy. Prior to undertaking definitive local therapy, especially radical prostatectomy (either by the perineal or retropubic route), it could be argued by some that the pelvic lymph nodes should be examined for the presence of metastatic cancer, since if the lymph nodes are found to be positive, it is generally considered a sign of disseminated disease and therefore a contraindication to pressing ahead with either form of extirpative prostatic surgery.

A further argument in favour of LPLND is that it permits lymph-node staging in individuals undergoing non-extirpative therapies (such as definitive external-beam radiotherapy) – especially those patients in studies where the results are being compared with those of surgery. Lack of staging data in the past has often skewed the results of radiation-therapy trials, and now this new, minimally invasive technique can facilitate more complete staging, allowing more valid comparisons between surgical and radiotherapeutic treatment options to be made. A description of the technique follows, based on that described by Sagalowsky and Preminger[19].

Creation of the pneumoperitoneum

In order to create the space within the peritoneal cavity for a LPLND to be accomplished, a pneumoperitoneum must be produced. This is usually achieved by the blind insertion of a Verress needle. These needles vary in length from 70 mm to 150 mm but the usual length in the adult is 120–150 mm. The needle consists of two components; a sharp outer bevelled sheath which houses an inner spring-loaded blunt tipped core. There is also a side attachment for insufflation of gas.

Selection of needle site

The inferior edge of the umbilicus is the most common site for the insertion of a Verress needle as it is the position where the distance between the skin and the peritoneum is least. It must be remembered, however, that in those patients with previous abdominal surgery, all needle and trocar sites must scrupulously

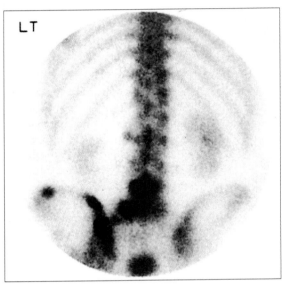 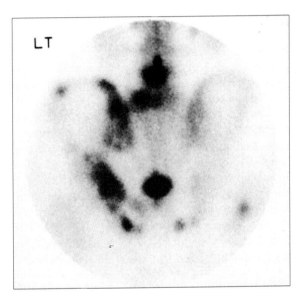

8.18 A strongly positive bone scan in a patient with metastatic prostate cancer: posterior spine (left), posterior pelvis (right).

Table 8.8 Correlation of serum PSA levels with radionuclide bone scan

PSA level (ng/ml)	Patients (%)	Positive scan (%)
0.0–4.0	89 (17)	0 (0)
4.1–10.0	118 (22)	0 (0)
10.1–20.0	99 (19)	1 (1)
20.1–50.0	99 (19)	7 (7)
50.1–100.0	60 (12)	23 (38)
> 100.0	56 (11)	40 (71)
TOTAL	521 (100)	71 (14)

(Chybowski et al., 1991[18])

avoid any areas related to previous incisions for fear of perforation of small or large bowel which may well be adherent to the anterior abdominal wall at this location. A semicircular skin incision is made within the lower edge of the umbilicus, care being taken to avoid inadvertent puncture of the peritoneum.

Technique of needle insertion

On pushing the Verress needle against the abdominal wall, the inner core automatically retracts, exposing the sharp outer sheath and it is this sheath that penetrates the rectus fascia. The anaesthetized patient is placed in a slight Trendelenburg position to allow intraperitoneal contents to fall away from the lower abdominal wall. A nasogastric tube and urethral catheter are inserted to keep both the bladder and stomach empty and thereby reduce the risks of inadvertent perforation of viscera. Whilst countertraction is applied to the infraumbilical skin, the Verress needle is introduced for a depth of 2–3 cm. The operator can often detect two distinct sensations of give as the needle goes first through the tough fascial layer and then through the peritoneal layer itself into the intra-abdominal space. Controlled but steady pressure is the best way to gain correct intraperitoneal placement. A slow twisting motion seems more likely to produce a faulty pre-peritoneal location of the instrument.

Confirmation of the needle position

Once the needle is in the peritoneal cavity, confirmatory tests must be performed prior to commencement of insufflation. Several means can be used to confirm the correct location of the Verress needle. The needle lumen should be free of any blood or fluid, and when a sterile 10 ml syringe primed with 5 ml of normal saline is attached, nothing should be retrieved. Aspiration of any coloured fluid, especially bowel content or gas, suggests injury to an underlying structure. If no fluid returns on aspiration, it is usually safe to inject a few millilitres of fluid into the abdominal cavity and attempt aspiration again. Fluid should immediately disperse through the intra-abdominal cavity, and therefore retrieval of the injected fluid should not be possible. If saline is reaspirated, the needle may be in a pocket formed by abdominal adhesions, or in a preperitoneal location; neither of these sites are appropriate for insufflation.

When a small needle puncture has been caused by the Verress needle placement, the injury can usually be managed conservatively. If however, there is any doubt about the degree of injury caused by the needle then serious consideration should be given to performing a mini-laparotomy to more fully assess the damage.

Insufflation

Once the operator is reasonably certain that the needle is in the correct intraperitoneal location, additional confirmation is obtained by connecting the insufflator to the needle. The initial intra-abdominal pressure should be low (less than 8 mmHg). Insufflation of carbon dioxide at a rate of 1 litre per minute should initially maintain intra-abdominal pressure of no more than 8 mmHg, a higher pressure than this suggests malposition of the needle and mandates replacement or reinsertion.

Once insufflation is safely underway, the abdomen should be monitored to ensure that a symmetrical, four quadrant pneumoperitoneum is developing. Loss of liver dullness should occur after insufflation of between 400 ml and 500 ml of gas.

The rate of insufflation of CO_2 may be gradually increased. Typically the highest setting on most insufflators is between 3 and 6 litres per minute; however the standard Verress needle will only allow about 2 litres per minute to flow due to the restrictive size of the lumen. Insufflation should continue until an intra-abdominal pressure of no more than 15 mmHg is reached. The usual adult requires between 4 and 5 litres of CO_2 for a full tense pneumoperitoneum to be accomplished. Once this is achieved, the Verress needle can be removed.

Trocar insertion

Both disposable and non-disposable trocar sheath units are now available from a variety of manufacturers. The non-disposable units are metallic and heavier than the disposable variety. Some sheaths have a roughened outer surface that helps grip the surrounding anterior abdominal wall. All trocar sheath units consist of two components, a hollow outer sheath and a sharp inner trocar housed within. The tip of the trocar is usually either pyramidal or conical, and easily penetrates through the anterio-abdominal wall layers. Once in the peritoneal cavity, the trocar is removed and the appropriate instrument may be passed down the sheath. The major advance in disposable trocar sheath technology has been the development of plastic safety shields which snap out to cover the trocar as it enters the pneumoperitoneum.

This shield retracts as pressure is applied, exposing the trocar tip. Once the trocar pierces the fascia the safety shield snaps forward and locks into position, thereby protecting the underlying bowel.

First trocar

The initial trocar employed is usually a 10 mm or 11 mm one, placed within the infraumbilical incision where the Verress needle was previously located. The incision needs to be sufficiently large for the trocar, yet tight enough around it to prevent loss of CO_2 during the procedure. Clearly, greater force is required to advance the 11 mm trocar through the fascia and peritoneum than is required for the much smaller Verress needle. Controlled insertion is even more important at this stage, to limit potentially dangerous intraperitoneal excursion of this sizeable instrument. In fact, the blind placement of the first trocar is probably the most hazardous point of the entire procedure.

In order to facilitate insertion of the first trocar without applying undue pressure, it may be helpful to incise the rectus fascia with a scalpel. The abdominal wall, tightly distended as a result of the pneumoperitoneum generally offers good counter pressure to the trocar so that rendering countertraction is unnecessary. The trocar is then advanced with a smooth steady pressure aimed perpendicularly to the fascia initially and then angled downwards to the hollow of the sacrum. Sometimes a twisting motion helps the tip of the instrument penetrate the fascia more easily.

Once the trocar-sheath unit is inserted at the umbilicus and the laparoscope camera applied, inspection of the underlying structures is undertaken to ensure that no injury has occurred and then the subsequent working ports can be established under laparoscopic monitoring.

Secondary trocars

The so-called diamond configuration of trocar insertion demonstrated in **8.19** is the one most commonly employed for LPLND. A 10 mm trocar is inserted in the midline, about 6 cm above the symphysis pubis, then two lateral 5 mm trocars are inserted in the left and right. Shining the light of the laparoscope intra-abdominally with the operating theatre lights turned down, sometimes helps delineate the superficial epigastric vessels which need to be avoided when these trocars are inserted. The lateral port should always be placed at the lateral border of the rectus and not through the rectus sheath to avoid the risk of significant bleeding.

The patient is then repositioned to the 30° Trendelenburg position with lateral rotation to allow loops of bowel to fall away from the iliac region of dissection.

Once the general survey of the abdomen is complete, the pelvic anatomy is assessed with the aim of identifying certain key pelvic landmarks. The peritoneal surface of the bladder is in the midline and with the urachus extending from the dome of the bladder to the umbilicus. The internal inguinal ring surrounds the spermatic cord and may be identified easily as it traverses the inferior pelvic side wall. The median umbilical ligament courses in an AP plane between the lateral wall of the bladder and the internal inguinal ring. The external iliac artery can be recognized beneath the peritoneum by its prominent pulsation. On the left side it is often necessary to take down adhesions of the sigmoid colon to achieve adequate access. On the right side both the caecum and the appendix may be tethered down over the iliac region and require gentle release.

The initial incision is accomplished through the posterior peritoneal membrane just lateral to the

Laparoscopic lymph node dissection

8.19 Positioning of trocars for laparoscopic pelvic lymph-node dissection.

obliterated umbilical artery (medial umbilical ligament) (**8.20a**). This incision provides entry into the obturator and iliac space. As the peritoneal incision is extended down into the pelvis the vas deferens comes into view crossing horizontally. This is a key structure in terms of orientation. The ureter, internal iliac artery and internal iliac vein are located just above and deep to the vas deferens. Any dissection above the vas therefore risks injury to these structures.

The lateral border of the lymphatic package is carefully freed by traction and countertraction, as succinctly described by Sagalowsky and Preminger[19], and dissected away from the external iliac artery. Subsequently the tissue is teased away from the more delicate and vulnerable external iliac vein. Not infrequently, an accessory obturator vein enters the external iliac vein from its medial aspect. This blood vessel should be secured and divided early to prevent avulsion during further mobilization of the lymph node package. It should be remembered that even a small amount of haemorrhage incurred during a laparoscopic procedure can markedly diminish visibility and make the procedure considerably more difficult.

At this stage in the procedure the lymph node package must be separated from the obturator nerve. Blunt dissection is utilized to identify this structure and the obturator artery and vein which are usually deep to it (**8.20a**). Once the tissue package is free, both medially and laterally, the remaining points of attachment are secured by clips: inferiorly near to the femoral canal and superiorly near the bifurcation of the internal and external iliac artery (**8.20b**). Careful clipping, especially inferiorly, minimizes the risk of subsequent lymphocoele development (**8.20b**). Once the specimen is completely free it can either be removed at this time or stored in an endoscopically placed bag for subsequent removal after the same manoeuvre has been completed on the other side. The lymphatic and fatty specimen is grasped with toothed forceps and thus withdrawn under direct vision. The patient is then rolled 20° upwards on the left and the procedure repeated on the contralateral side.

Once the operation is complete and the lymphatic tissue from both obturator fossae successfully removed, the pelvis should be irrigated with heparinized saline solution (5000 units/l) and carefully checked for bleeding. To complete the operation the trocars are sequentially removed under direct vision, remembering that the first trocar site was established blindly, and is therefore the most likely source of unde-

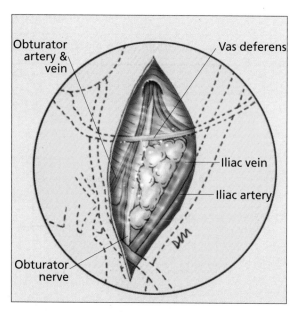

8.20(a) Laparoscopic view of the obturator lymph nodes. The overlying peritoneum is incised. (Modified with permission from Sagalowsky and Preminger[19].)

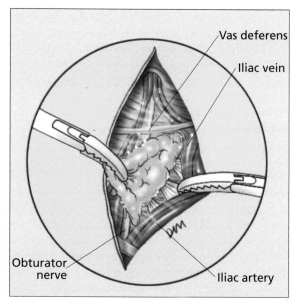

(b) The package of tissue is carefully dissected away from the obturator nerve and vessels and the external iliac vein and lymph nodes removed for histological assessment. (Modified with permission from Sagalowsky and Preminger[19].)

tected bleeding. Finally the pneumoperitoneum is evacuated as completely as possible to reduce post-operative pain and distension and the patient is returned to the recovery area.

Results

The technique is new and few comparative data are as yet available. Schuessler et al.[20] reported their experience with transperitoneal endosurgical lymphadenectomy with patients with localized prostate cancer. Twelve patients underwent LPLND for staging prior to percutaneous radioactive-seed implantation for prostate cancer. The operative time ranged from 90–205 minutes; an average of 7.6 nodes were removed from the right obturator fossa and 7.1 from the left. No procedure was converted to an open lymphadenectomy and there were no post-operative patients. The mean hospital stay was only 1 day. Parra and co-workers[21] randomized 24 men to either open or laparoscopic lymphadenectomy and found similar yields in terms of lymphatic tissue, but a lesser morbidity for the laparoscopic method. Troxel and Winfield[22] found that although the total costs were greater for LPLND than for open lymph node removal, these extra costs were more than justified by the rapid return to normal activity.

CONCLUSIONS

Accurate staging of prostate cancer is important in selecting the proper form of therapy. DRE, PSA testing, TRUS, CT and MRI scanning all have a role, but understaging and overstaging remain frequent clinical problems. The advantages of LPLND lie in its accuracy in terms of confirming or refuting lymph-node involvement, and in the short hospital stay. However, since only a small proportion of patients undergoing radical prostatectomy are now found to have positive lymph nodes (and nearly always in patients with larger volume, higher-stage tumours with significantly raised PSA values), it seems logical to restrict LPLND to that category of case. This should reduce what would otherwise be an unacceptably large proportion of cases in whom the lymph nodes would subsequently be found, on histological evaluation, to be negative. Whether this rather time-consuming and technically demanding technique will be widely taken up by urologists worldwide remains to be seen.

For more complete reviews of the LPLND technique, the reader is referred to the recent publications of Sagalowsky and Preminger[19] and Gomella, Kozminski and Winfield[23].

REFERENCES

1. Spigelman SS, McNeal JE, Freiha FS, et al. Rectal examination in volume determination of carcinoma of the prostate: clinical and anatomical correlations. J Urol 1986;**136**:1228–1230.
2. Bosch RJLH, Kurth KH, Schroder FH. Surgical treatment of locally advanced (T3) prostatic carcinoma: early results. J Urol, 1987;**138**:816–822.
3. Littrup PJ, Williams CR, Egglin TK. Determination of prostate volume with transrectal ultrasound for cancer screening II. Radiology, 1991;**179**:49–53.
4. Rifkin MD (1988) Prostate cancer sonographic characteristics. In: Ultrasound of the Prostate. Rifkin MD (Ed). Raven Press, New York, p 179.
5. Scardino PT, Shinohara K, Wheeler TM, et al. Staging of prostate cancer: value of ultrasonography. Urologic Clinics of N America, 1989;**16**:713–734.
6. Ohori M, Egawa S, Shinohara K, et al.. Detection of microscopic extra-capsular extension prior to radical prostatectomy for clinically localised prostate cancer. Br J Urol, 1994;**74**:72–79.
7. Narayan P, Jajodia P, Stein R. Core biopsy instrument in the diagnosis of prostate cancer superior accuracy to fine needle aspiration. J Urol, 1991;**145**:795–799.
8. Gammelgaard J, Holm HH. Trans-urethral and trans-rectal ultrasound scanning in urology. J Urol, 1980;**124**,863–868.
9. Platt JF, Bree RL, Schwab RE. The accuracy of CT in the staging of carcinoma of the prostate. Am J Radiol, 1987;**149**:315–318.
10. Sukov RJ, Scardino PT, Sample WF, et al. Computed tomography and trans-abdominal ultrasound in the evaluation of the prostate. J Computer Assisted Tomography, 1977;**1**:281–289.
11. Bryan PJ, Butler HE, Nelson AD, et al. Magnetic resonance imaging of the prostate. Am J Radiol, 1986;**146**: 543–548.
12. Hricak H, Dooms GC, Jeffrey RB, et al. Prostatic carcinoma: staging by clinical assessment, CT and MRI imaging. Radiol, 1987;**162**:331–336.
13. Rifkin MD, Zerlouri EA, Gatsonis CA, et al. Comparison of magnetic resonance imaging and ultrasonography in staging early prostate cancer. New Eng J Med 1990;**323**: 621–625.

14. Schnall MD, Imai Y, Tomaszewski J, *et al.*. Prostate cancer: local staging with endorectal surface coil MR imaging. *Radiol*, 1991;**178**:797–802.

15. Loening SA, Schmidt JD, Brown RC, *et al.* A comparison between lymphangiography and pelvic node dissection in the staging of prostatic cancer. J *Urol*, 1977;**117**:752–756.

16. O'Mara RE. Skeletal scanning in neoplastic disease. *Cancer*, 1977;**37**:480–486.

17. Miller PD, Eardley I, Kirby RS. Prostate specific antigen and bone scan correlation in staging and monitoring of patients with prostate cancer. Br J *Urol*, 1992;**70**:295–298.

18. Chybowski FM, Larson Keller JJ, Bergstralh EJ, *et al.* Predicting radionucleotide bone scan findings in patients with newly diagnosed untreated prostate cancer: prostate specific antigen is superior to all other parameters. J *Urol*, 1991;**145**:313–318.

19. Sagalowsky AI, Preminger GM. *Basic Urologic Laparoscopy* Futura Publishing Co Inc, New York 1993:110–111

20. Schuessler W, Vancaillie TG, Reich H, *et al.* Transperitoneal endosurgical lymphadenectomy in patients with localized prostate cancer. J *Urol*. 1991;**145**:988–991.

21. Parra RO, Andrus C, Boullier J. Staging laparoscopic pelvic lymph node dissection: comparison of results with open pelvic lymphadenectomy. J *Urol* 1992;**147**:875–878.

22. Troxel S, Winfield HN. Comparative financial analysis of laparoscopic versus open pelvic lymph node dissection for men with cancer of the prostate. J *Urol* 1994;**151**:675–680.

23. Gomella GL, Kozminski M, Winfield HN. *Laparoscopic Urologic Surgery* Raven Press, New York, 1994, 111–130

CHAPTER 9
TREATMENT OF LOCALIZED PROSTATE CANCER: RADICAL PROSTATECTOMY AND RADIATION THERAPY

The treatment of clinically localized adenocarcinoma of the prostate has undergone considerable evolution and refinement over the 90 years that have passed since Hugh Hampton Young developed the radical perineal prostatectomy (**Table 9.1**). Factors such as downward stage migration in the clinical presentation, the development of and subsequent improvements in radiation delivery to the prostate, as well as modifications in surgical technique associated with decreased morbidity, have all contributed towards enhancement in treatment approaches for confined prostate cancer.

Implicit within the concept of treatment of clinically localized cancer is the ability to identify such cancers at a stage where effective therapy is both possible and necessary.

The determination of a localized malignancy (T1–T3) is dependent upon accurate staging techniques. As discussed in the chapter on staging, one of the major problems in prostate cancer is our inability to define the clinical stage precisely. Significant up-staging and, to a lesser degree, downstaging of neoplasms in men subjected to radical prostatectomy

have consistently demonstrated the inadequacy of current staging modalities[1-7]. Currently, urologists use DRE, serum acid phosphatase and prostate specific antigen and transrectal ultrasound techniques, as well as other methods including computed tomography, magnetic resonance imaging and, more recently, endorectal coil magnetic resonance imaging, to assist in arriving at the clinical stage.

The use of prostate specific antigen in combination with clinical stage and Gleason score on biopsy has been shown by the Johns Hopkins group to improve the ability to predict pathological stage as compared to each variable independently[8]. These authors have provided nomograms to predict pathological stage. However, it should be noted that this series derives from a highly selected patient cohort of men with generally well-differentiated, small-volume prostate cancer, treated in a single institution.

The use of tissue-derived parameters to augment staging studies, including tumour grade, DNA ploidy and investigational studies of neovascularity, expression of oncogenes and tumour suppressor genes, as

Table 9.1 Milestones in the treatment of prostate cancer

Year	Author	Milestone
1904	Young	Development of radical prostatectomy
1910	Paschkis, Tittinger	Intraurethral radium
1934	Widmann	External beam radiation
1941	Huggins, Hodges	Hormonal ablation
1979	Wang	Characterization of PSA
1979	Reiner, Walsh	Anatomical radical prostatectomy
1982	Walsh, Donker	Nerve sparing radical prostatectomy
1987	Labrie	Maximal androgen blockade

well as growth factors, is discussed more fully in the chapters on molecular biology and pathology.

With the increasing worldwide interest in early detection and screening, there has been a pronounced movement towards a more favourable stage at presentation (both between stages in general, and within given stages), which is most marked in the USA. Instead of the bulky T3/T4 cancers with gross capsular penetration and extension into the pelvic sidewall or seminal vesicles, most modern radical prostatectomy series currently describe only minimal, microscopic capsular penetration or positive margins in patients who are pathologically upstaged. Thus, it is not always appropriate to apply the lessons of historical series to current patient care.

The goal of treatment of clinically localized prostate cancer is cure; that is to say, as suggested by a recent prostate cancer consensus meeting in Antwerp, Belgium[9], 'affording the patient the best chance of dying of something else'. A number of factors need to be considered when deciding whether a patient is suitable for therapy with curative intent. Perhaps of greatest significance is that the patient should have at least a ten-year life expectancy. Thus, an accurate assessment of intercurrent disease, as well as other risk factors for longevity, must be conducted. As the majority of men with clinically localized prostate cancer will have minimal impact from their disease for several years at least, it obviously makes little sense to subject an individual to the morbidity of locally directed therapy if they have a truncated life expectancy.

The treatment options (**Table 9.2**) include watchful waiting or expectant management, radical prostatectomy, radiation therapy delivered by either external or brachytherapy approaches, androgen deprivation and, more recently, cryotherapeutic ablation. It should be noted at the outset that a major problem in our understanding and evaluation of these alternative treatment modalities is the lack of adequate long-term randomized trials to compare and contrast the merits of one therapy with another. In the absence of such studies, it is exceedingly difficult to offer answers as to which treatment modality is optimal for a given individual.

Another difficulty in evaluating the different treatment modalities is the problem inherent in defining what is 'cure'. **Table 9.3** illustrates a hierarchical schema of the evidence of failure of cure in prostate cancer. Given that the goal of treatment of clinically localized prostate cancer is to afford the opportunity of the patient to die of something else, one might conclude that patients are 'cured' if this is achieved.

However, even in this simplistic approach, confusion arises as it is often difficult to state definitively whether a patient with prostate cancer actually died of his disease. Given the age of the patients at risk with significant intercurrent illness, competing causes of mortality must always be considered in the aetiology of a patient's demise. However, even in cases of clear-cut progression of disease, one must consider whether 'failed' local therapy actually afforded improvement in the patient's quality and quantity of life.

Table 9.2 Localized prostate cancer: therapeutic options
Watchful waiting
Transurethral resection
Radical prostatectomy
External-beam radiation therapy
Brachytherapy
Cryotherapy
Androgen deprivation
Laser combination therapy
Interstitial laser therapy

Table 9.3 Possible definitions of cure
Death from non-prostatic cause
Absence of disseminated disease
Absence of local/regional disease
Negative prostate or prostatic bed biopsy
Normal rectal examination
Non-detectable serum PSA

This concept is certainly biased by the development of a valuable marker of progression of prostate cancer – prostate specific antigen (PSA). This analyte, particularly in men following radical prostatectomy, affords absolute and unequivocal evidence of progression in that, if the PSA does fall to the non-detectable level, then there is evidence of persistent disease, and if PSA falls but subsequently becomes detectable at ever higher levels, there is progression. PSA is an exquisitely sensitive marker of progression, and is generally a harbinger of subsequent clinical disease. One can therefore rely on this simple assay to select patients for further evaluation of potential of progression, including radionucleotide bone scan for bony metastases, upper tract studies to assess hydronephrosis, serum creatinine, and full blood count to assess systemic illness, and so forth.

However, whether this biochemical evidence of progression actually indicates a deterioration in the patients' quality and quantity of life is not known. Certainly, a man who has a detectable level of PSA 12 years after radical prostatectomy has evidence of persistent disease. If he succumbs to a myocardial infarction, it would seem that his persistent disease contributed little to his demise. Thus one could argue in pragmatic terms that he was 'cured'.

PSA allows us to monitor patients following radical prostatectomy with greater reliability. Its use after radiation therapy remains somewhat confusing, however, but it seems highly likely that progressive elevation of PSA as well as failure to achieve a significant nadir after definitive radiation therapy are ominous prognostic indicators.

In general, with either of these treatment approaches, PSA monitoring in conjunction with history and physical examination provides the most efficient and economical approach to following patients after therapy. None the less, it has to be conceded that patients run a risk of becoming 'self obsessed' by their PSA result, regardless of whether a PSA rise is in fact accompanied by symptoms.

RADICAL PROSTATECTOMY

Radical prostatectomy has been recommended by some for almost all stages of prostate cancer. Affording cure is the goal in localized disease, whereas efforts to provide a reduction in local symptoms of progression is the intent in patients with established, advanced disease. Radical prostatectomy is widely used today only in men in whom it is likely to afford cure – in effect, only in those in whom it is felt that the malignancy is completely extirpable by surgery. This, in general, applies to those men with a stage T1 or T2 disease with low-to-moderate grade pathology and a life expectancy of more than 10 years. Cure may be achieved in some patients with minimal T3 disease, and perhaps a very few with minimal lymph node metastases. **Table 9.4** depicts the criteria for the selection of patients for radical prostatectomy.

Patients undergoing radical retropubic prostatectomy should be evaluated with a careful history and physical examination, with care being taken to detect comorbidity due to underlying cardiovascular and pulmonary disease. Chest x-ray and electrocardiography, along with urinalysis, serum creatinine and complete blood count, are obtained. Many surgeons now ask the patients to donate 2–3 units of autologous blood prior to the procedure. A cleansing enema and systemic antimicrobial prophylaxis are used.

The goal of radical prostatectomy, whether by the retropubic or perineal approach, is to achieve complete excision of the prostate, seminal vesicles and adjacent tissue. The caudal and cephalad margins include the membranous urethra and the bladder neck. The posterior margin is Denonvillier's fascia, and anteriorly is the fibroadipose tissue of the cave of Retzius. Laterally, the boundary is the prostatic plexus medial to the neurovascular bundle if a nerve-sparing approach is performed.

Radical retropubic prostatectomy can now be reliably accomplished in less than 2–3 hours with minimal morbidity. The patient is placed on the operating table with 10–20° of break at its midpoint to increase the distance between the pubis and xiphisternum. A 22F urethral catheter is passed and balloon inflated. A lower-midline abdominal incision is made and the dissection kept extraperitoneal. Bilateral, internal iliac node dissections are performed (if these have not been accomplished

Table 9.4 Criteria for radical prostatectomy

Histological evidence of prostate cancer

Clinically localized stage T1–T2

10-year or more life expectancy

Absence of surgical contraindication

Adequate informed consent

beforehand by LPLND), and frozen section histology obtained (if there is reasonable degree of suspicion that they may be positive, i.e. PSA >10 ng/ml).

Attention is then paid to the division of the avascular puboprostatic ligaments close to the pubis (**9.1**), and to securing the dorsal venous complex. If this is accomplished successfully, blood loss from the entire procedure rarely exceeds 750–1000 ml. After 'bunching' the structure with a long-handled Babcock retractor (**9.2**), a strong absorbable ligature or suture may be

passed around the dorsal vein complex, which is then divided to expose the urethra, as it enters the apex of the prostate. Careful dissection in this location using a Gil-Vernet renal retractor increases the length of urethra for subsequent anastomosis to the bladder neck. The urethra and the catheter it contains are then divided sharply, with careful attention being paid to the avoidance of the neurovascular bundles, which are located dorsolaterally (but very close to the apex of the prostate) at this point. The proximal end of the catheter

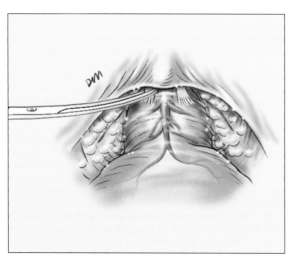

9.1 The puboprostatic ligaments are divided near to the pubis.

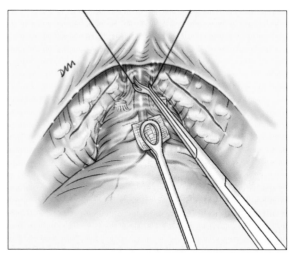

9.2 The dorsal venous complex is 'bunched' with a long-handled Babcock retractor.

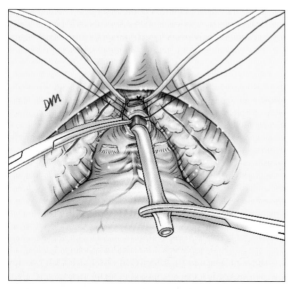

9.3 The anterior aspect of the urethra is sharply divided, the catheter cut, and its proximal end used as a retractor. The posterior portion is then divided.

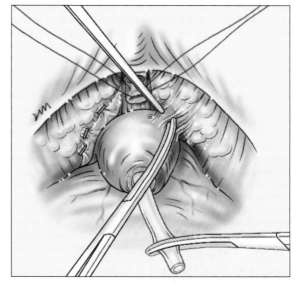

9.4 The lateral pedicles containing vessels are clipped and divided close to the prostate, thus preserving the neurovascular bundles.

may then be used as a retractor to facilitate the 'peeling back' of the prostate with the division of the rest of the urethra (**9.3**), and the stepwise securement and division of the lateral vascular pedicles, keeping close to the prostate to preserve the internally placed neurovascular bundles (**9.4**). The seminal vesicles and ampullary portions of both vasa come into view, and may be dissected out via this inferior approach. The ampullary portions of both vasa are divided, and the seminal vesicles freed (**9.5**). The prostate is then care-

fully dissected away from the bladder neck, using a bladder-neck sparing technique (**9.6**). The catheter is then used as a loop retractor to facilitate dissection of the junction of the trigone and the prostate (**9.7**), and the specimen plus the seminal vesicles are removed. After eversion of the bladder mucosa to prevent anastomotic stricture an anastomosis is created between the bladder neck and urethra over a 20F urethral catheter using from four to seven absorbable Vicryl or Dexon sutures (**9.8**). A corrugated wound drain is

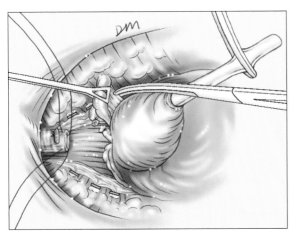

9.5 The ampullary portion of each vas is divided and the seminal vesicles dissected free, their apical vessels having been clipped.

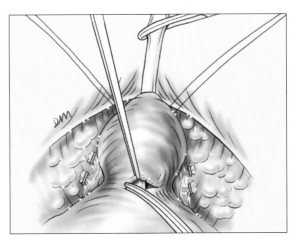

9.6 The prostate is carefully dissected away from the bladder neck.

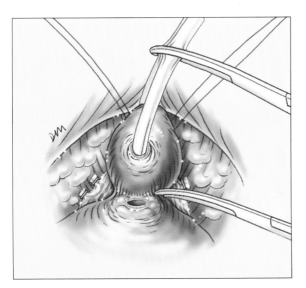

9.7 The catheter is used as a 'loop retractor' to help the separation of the prostate from the trigone.

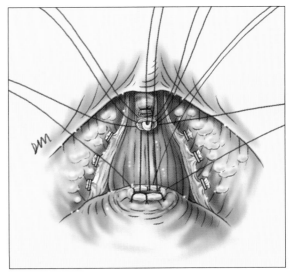

9.8 An anastomosis is created with 4–7 absorbable sutures between the bladder neck with its everted mucosa and urethra.

inserted and the wound closed in layers.

Early post-operative mobilization is encouraged, free fluids started the first post-operative day, and most patients leave hospital on the sixth post-operative day. The urethral catheter is retained for two to three weeks and, on its removal, most patients are fully continent.

Table 9.5 demonstrates the advantages and disadvantages of radical prostatectomy. Clearly the greatest advantage of this treatment is that, if indeed the cancer is 'specimen confined', the patient may be generally assured of cure (**9.9**). This allays significant anxiety in the post-operative period – a factor of considerable importance in this neoplasm given the long natural history. Significant advances in surgical technique, pioneered by Walsh and associates at Johns Hopkins, Baltimore, USA, have made the operation considerably safer, with reduction of blood loss and decrease in significant urinary incontinence[10,11]. Moreover, when a nerve sparing approach is elected, preservation of potency in at least a proportion of younger men may be achieved[12-15]. Finally, radical prostatectomy affords the benefit of definitive treatment of bladder-outlet obstruction owing to benign prostatic hyperplasia – a condition frequently co-affecting patients diagnosed with carcinoma.

There are, however, a number of disadvantages to radical prostatectomy. This is still a not inconsiderable operation, with potential for morbidity and indeed occasional mortality. The latter has been shown to be low in a large US series (**Table 9.6**). However, more widespread application of this surgical procedure has resulted in reports of higher mortality rates[16].

Damage to surrounding structures, namely the ureter and rectum, may occur during the surgical procedure. However, in general, if these are recognized and repaired, with the judicious employment of an omental wrap during the operative procedure, there are few long-term side-effects.

Major long-term complications include urethral strictures, incontinence and erectile dysfunction. The frequency of urethral stricture is about 5% or less and, in general, is relatively easily handled. The treatment of problematic strictures, however, may sometimes render the patient incontinent.

Urinary incontinence has been reduced significantly by the development of an anatomical approach to radical retropubic prostatectomy. Nevertheless, incontinence still can and does occur and, in general, some troublesome incontinence may be expected to be seen in approximately 3% of patients. Major or total incontinence requiring the placement of an artificial urinary sphincter or, more recently, the injection of collagen (Bard Urologic, Covington, GA, USA) is now unusual. Recently, Herr[17] evaluated the impact of urinary incontinence in men undergoing radical prostatectomy. He noted that whereas 74% dealt well with their morbid-

Table 9.5 Advantages and disadvantages of radical prostatectomy

Advantages	Disadvantages
Cure if pathologically confined	Major operation
Definitive staging	Potential mortality
Treatment of symptomatic BPH	Potential morbidity including:
Decreased patient anxiety in follow-up	impotence,
Ease of monitoring for persistent	incontinence,
disease	rectal injury,
	urethral stricture,
	bleeding
	May not be necessary

ity with no limitations in activities, 26% were significantly bothered. A total of 64% of the men stated that if asked to decide on therapy again they would again choose surgery.

Erectile dysfunction previously occurred in virtually 100% of patients undergoing radical prostatectomy. The recognition of pelvic plexus innervation of the corpora cavernosa has allowed sparing of the nerves and the maintenance of erectile function in a significant percentage of men[12-15]. Risk factors for failure of this approach include patient age, pre-operative sexual function level, tumour stage, and, perhaps most importantly, the surgeon's experience. Sacrifice of the nerve ipsilateral to the clinically recognized cancer, while reducing somewhat the potency rate, still affords maintenance of erection in many individuals, with perhaps some decrease in the rate of positive margins, as compared with a bilateral nerve sparing approach.

Little data are available with regard to a definitive evaluation of sexual function prior to and after a radical retropubic prostatectomy. Such studies are certainly indicated for our greater understanding of the adequacy of erection and sexual function in general in men so treated. It is interesting to note, however, that in our experience in the US and the UK, a relatively small percentage of men seek active treatment of erectile dysfunction following radical prostatectomy. Of those that do, the majority respond well to intracavernous pharmacotherapy using papaverine or more recently prostaglandin E1.

Other complications of radical prostatectomy may include thrombophlebitis and pulmonary emboli, development of a lymphocoele, anastomotic urinary leakage, and wound infection.

Radical prostatectomy may be performed by two alternative surgical approaches: either retropubic as described, or perineal. The perineal was the first approach to be used, and has certain advantages to the retropubic, including probably fewer complications in the post-operative period, particularly in patients with pulmonary disease. Decreased blood loss and ease of performing the vesico-urethral anastomosis are also claimed. One particular disadvantage of this

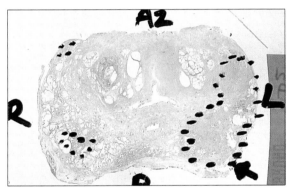

9.9 A whole mount specimen showing a sizable tumour in the left peripheral zone and a smaller cancer in the right peripheral zone. Both cancers were specimen confined.

Table 9. 6 Pelvic lymphadenectomy and radical retropubic prostatectomy operative mortality rate 1982–1992				
Institution	Dates	Total No. Patients	No. of Deaths	Mortality Rate (%)
Baylor	1988–92	764	2	0.26
Washington University	1983–92	810	0	0
Johns Hopkins	1982–92	1300	2	0.15
Stanford	1984–92	700	0	0
Total		3574	4	0.11
After Scardino, presented at the American Urological Association Meeting, 1993, San Antonio				

technique is the inability to perform a pelvic lymph-node dissection. However, this may be provided by a prior pelvic lymphadenectomy achieved by either open or laparoscopic technique (see Chapter 8). Recently, Levy and Resnick[18] have described the use of radical perineal prostatectomy following laparoscopic pelvic lymphadenectomy as a viable option.

Technique of Radical Perineal Prostatectomy

The following description of radical perineal prostatectomy is based on the excellent and more complete reviews by Vernon E. Weldon in *Prostate Cancer* (Marcel Dekker, New York, 1993) and that of David F. Paulson

in *Prostate Diseases* (WB Saunders, Philadelphia, 1993). The procedure is undertaken with the patient in the exaggerated lithotomy position. An inverted U-shaped incision is then made as shown in **9.10**. Deepening of this incision is accomplished by careful transection of the central muscles of the perineum which connect the external anal sphincter to the transverse perineal and

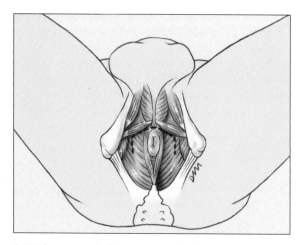

9.10 The anatomical structures underlying the U-shaped perineal incision (dotted line) for radical perineal prostatectomy. (Modified with permission from Weldon[79].)

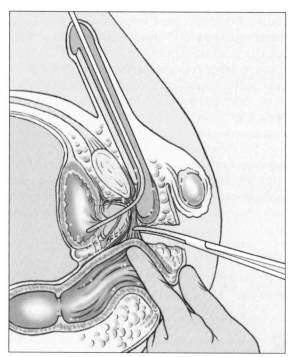

9.11 A curved urethral tractor puts the rectourethralis muscle on the stretch. (Modified with permission from Weldon[79].)

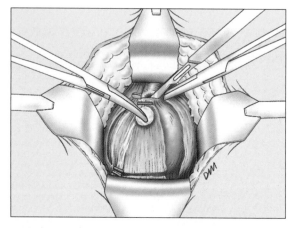

9.12 The posterior aspect of the urethra is divided under direct vision at the apex of the prostate. (Modified with permission from Weldon[79].)

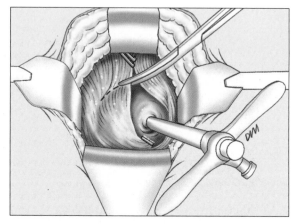

9.13 A short, straight prostatic tractor helps to mobilize the prostate and facilitates division of the lateral pedicles close to the gland. (Modified with permission from Weldon[79].)

bulbospongiosus muscles at the perineal body. The rectal sphincter can then be visualized as a muscular arch overlying the rectum. Dissection beneath this musculature reveals the pale anterior rectal fascia which serves as a guide to the prostate.

At this point, or a little earlier, it is helpful to insert a prostatic tractor retrogradely into the bladder. The Loseley curved tractor is often easier to insert than the Young's straight prostatic tractor. If there is difficulty inserting either of these devices then a urethral catheter or urethral sound may be used (**9.11**). Identification of the rectourethralis muscle is assisted by placing it under tension. The rectum is tented upwards by the muscle, and therefore division of these muscle fibres permits posterior displacement of the rectum. At this stage identification of the rectum can be facilitated by the insertion of a finger in it, a manoeuvre that may prevent inadvertant damage to the structure. Blunt dissection then permits the exposure of the lateral anterior margins of the prostate. The overlying prostatic fascia appears white and glistening and should usually be removed intact with the specimen. If, however, a potently preserving prostatectomy is intended, this structure can be divided in the midline so that the periprostatic neurovascular plexi can be preserved on one or both sides.

The membranous urethra is then exposed at the prostatic apex and gently freed from its surrounding tissues and encircled using a right-angled clamp. The dorsal wall of the membranous urethra is transected sharply just at its junction with the prostatic apex (**9.12**). The incision is then carried down to the pro-

static tractor or catheter which is removed, and the ventral urethral wall is transected.

At this stage, a short straight prostatic tractor is passed through the prostatic urethra into the bladder and the blades extended. The presence of this device helps to mobilize the prostate and facilitates dissection and division of the lateral pedicles close to the gland (**9.13**). The lateral prostatic fascia usually contains several large vessels, and it is often helpful to place haemostatic clips systematically along these fascial sheaths and transect beneath the clips. Rotation of the straight prostatic tractor contralaterally exposes the remaining lateral prostatic fascia which can then be transected up to the level of the bladder neck. Anterior bladder neck transection can then be accomplished with careful preservation of the circular detrusor fibres which may be separated by careful dissection from the prostate, exposing the bladder neck mucosa. At this stage, it is often helpful to withdraw the Young's straight prostatic tractor and replace it with a Foley catheter, which can be passed through the prostatic urethra and brought out as a loop superiorly through the line of the incision between the prostate and the bladder neck. Traction on this catheter permits the prostate to be displaced posteriorly and defines the line of cleavage between the bladder neck and the prostate.

The posterior vesical neck musculature can then be divided sharply in the midline down to the anterior fascia overlying the ampulla of the vasa differentia and seminal vesicles. As in radical retropubic prostatectomy, the posterior bladder neck muscle is often found to be quite thick and this dissection therefore needs to be continued deeper than is often anticipated. In both radical retropubic and perineal prostatectomy, dissection in the wrong plane runs a risk of inadvertent injury to the ureters. In the circumstance of the plane of transection being unclear, it is often safer to delay this dissection until the time of division of the vascular pedicles when the seminal vesicles, ampullary portions of the vasa and the plane of the genital fascia are easier to visualize (**9.14**). At this stage the prostate and seminal vesicles remain secured posterio-laterally by the vascular pedicles, but the entire gland is free from the bladder.

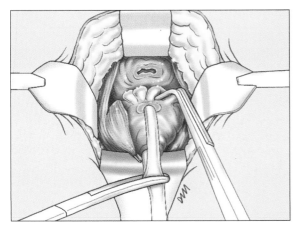

9.14 The seminal vesicles and ampullary portions of the vasa are dissected free and the vasa divided. (Modified with permission from Weldon[79].)

The vascular pedicles can be isolated at 5 and 7 o'clock, and controlled either by surgical clips or by the careful insertion of absorbable sutures. After division of these pedicles bilaterally, the specimen is then held only by the seminal vesicles and the vasa deferentia. The vasa deferentia may be clipped and divided.

Often small blood vessels are found at the apex of the seminal vesicles and these should be controlled either by diathermy or by the use of clips before the entire specimen is removed and sent for pathological examination.

Once reasonable haemostasis has been accomplished, reconstruction of the bladder neck is often necessary. The anterior bladder neck is then anastomosed to the membranous urethra using 4 to 7 absorbable sutures over a 20 or 22F silicone Foley catheter (**9.15**). Further sutures may be inserted into the bladder neck as this anastomosis is accomplished so that the bladder neck is snug around the catheter. The wound is then closed in layers with a corrugated drain left down to the anastomosis, and the U-shaped skin incision repaired using either an interrupted or a subcuticular absorbable suture (**9.16**). Early postoperative mobilisation is encouraged and the catheter generally retained for a period of about two weeks, but the patient is often able to leave hospital within 72 hours of surgery.

Efficacy of Radical Prostatectomy

Most urologists today favour retropubic rather than perineal radical prostatectomy. This is largely due to the familiarity with the retropubic anatomy, but also because this approach affords the opportunity for wider excision of adjacent tissue in patients who may have extension of their neoplasm through the capsule.

Moreover, a pelvic lymphadenectomy may be readily performed, rapidly, and with minimal morbidity through the same incision. This provides definitive staging and inherent prognostic information, but the therapeutic benefit of lymphadenectomy itself has never been demonstrated.

As noted, it is difficult to make meaningful conclusions about the outcome of treatment owing to a number of factors. The significant competing mortalities, along with the variable natural history of prostatic carcinoma, mandate long-term follow-up prior to making definitive conclusions with regard to cure. Several studies of long-term follow-up are available (**Table 9.7**), demonstrating excellent overall mortality which compares favourably to age-matched controls without prostatic carcinoma.

It should be emphasized that these earlier series involved profiles different from those of patients generally operated on today. Significant stage migration, improvements in staging techniques and more accurate grading strategies now allow more appropriate selection of patients for radical prostatectomy than in the historical series. In many of the older series, radionucleotide bone scans were not performed and, as the majority of these patients underwent perineal prostatectomy, definitive nodal staging afforded by pelvic lymphadenectomy was not provided. It would seem likely that, owing to these differences, and the important influence of PSA measurement plus improved surgical

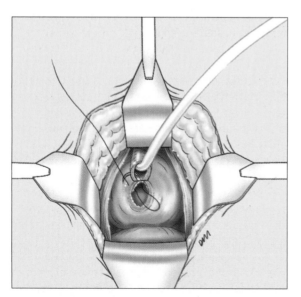

9.15 The urethra and bladder neck are anastomosed with interrupted sutures over a catheter. (Modified with permission from Weldon[79].)

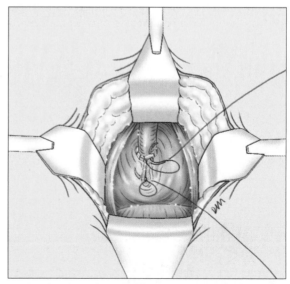

9.16 The anastomosis is completed with a closure of the bladder neck itself. (Modified with permission from Weldon[79].)

techniques, more contemporary series will provide even better disease-free survival outcomes.

The reduction in morbidity afforded by the anatomical approach to radical prostatectomy has resulted in some surgeons extending the indication to men with clinical T3 disease. There has been renewed interest in upfront (neoadjuvant) hormonal-deprivation therapy to shrink and hopefully downstage the tumour in patients with clinical T3 disease prior to radical prostatectomy. While definitive answers cannot be provided, Labrie *et al.* demonstrated significant reduction in positive margins in men receiving three months of an antiandrogen plus an LHRH agonist prior to radical prostatectomy, when compared to men undergoing immediate surgery without hormone therapy[19]. Other studies, while demonstrating significant reduction in serum PSA and tumour size, have rarely shown actual downstaging to organ-confined disease. Randomized trials applying neoadjuvant hormonal manipulation are underway in the USA and in Europe, and definitive answers will soon be provided.

The inadequacies of current pre-operative staging procedures noted above have resulted in considerable pathological upstaging (**9.15**) in men undergoing radical prostatectomy to capsular penetration or beyond. **Table 9.8** demonstrates the incidence of this in several series.

The identification of pathological upstaging (capsular extension, positive margins, seminal vesicle extension, etc.) is certainly intrinsically related to the thoroughness of the pathological examination of the surgical specimen. Even with rigorous step sectioning, the detection of cancer cells dotted with ink on the margin of the specimen may not provide definitive evidence that residual neoplasm is left within the patient. In this regard, post-operative serum PSA is particularly helpful. An 'iatrogenic' margin owing to traumatic denuding of the prostatic capsule may result in a false positive margin. Each laboratory must determine their lower limit of detectability of serum PSA and, in general, one should not make therapeutic decisions until a trend of increasing PSA above this nadir level is noted.

In the face of detectable serum PSA post-operatively, the next step should be an attempt at determining whether this is owing to residual local disease or whether it represents systemic carcinoma. Review of the pathological report may help in this regard, and, if a positive margin is noted this suggests that there may be local disease; however, this certainly does not exclude systemic cancer. Men who have positive seminal vesicles and particularly those with positive pelvic lymph nodes may, in general, be assumed to have disseminated disease. A radionucleotide bone scan in

Table 9.7 Radical prostatectomy 15-year NED* and survival

Author	Clinical stage	Pathological stage	No.	15-year NED/survival
Jewett[30]	B1	B–C2	86	28 (33)
	B1	C3	17	0
Elder[7]	B2	B	14	7 (50)
	B2	C2–3	32	4 (13)
Gibbons[6]	B1	B,C	43	26 (61)
	B2	B,C	9	3 (33)

* NED = No evidence of disease

Table 9.8 Incidence of extracapsular disease after radical prostatectomy

Author	Clin. Stage	No.	No. upstaged (%)
Lange[1]	A2	6	3 (50)
Boxer[2]	A	35	8 (23)
Catalona[3]	A2	9	1 (11)
Veenema[4]	A,B	159	66 (42)
Jewett[5]	B1	103	26 (25)
Catalona[3]	B1	48	8 (17)
Gibbons[6]	B	143	46 (31)
Lange[1]	B2	25	15 (60)
Catalona[3]	B2	23	9 (39)
Elder[7]	B2	53	35 (66)

this setting is imperative and, if a pre-operative scan was obtained, the prior study must be carefully compared to the subsequent examination. Magnetic resonance or plain x-ray imaging of equivocal bone scan findings may improve specificity. Pelvic imaging studies in this setting have in general been unsatisfactory in detecting low levels of persistent clinical disease. Some authorities[20] have reported on digitally guided biopsy of the region of the vesical–urethral anastomosis to define pelvic disease persistence. The use of transrectal ultrasound alone has in general been disappointing in the demonstration of residual neoplasm[21].

Table 9.9 describes the incidence of clinical evidence of local recurrence after radical prostatectomy. If it is felt that the patient is at risk for local recurrence owing to the pathological stage, particularly if PSA is detectable following radical prostatectomy, many authorities recommend adjuvant radiation therapy.

Table 9.10 illustrates several reports demonstrating a significantly decreased local recurrence rate in men treated with adjuvant radiation therapy. While most studies have observed this, the absence of the randomized prospective data makes attempts at definitive conclusions unwarranted. Long-term follow-up with regard to cancer-specific and all-cause mortality in patients receiving adjuvant therapy is also lacking.

Currently, trials evaluating both adjuvant hormonal therapy and radiation therapy in this setting are underway.

Adjuvant radiation therapy certainly contributes somewhat to morbidity. However, it is generally well-tolerated if it is delayed until the maximum return of urinary incontinence, if a limited pelvic lymphadenectomy has been performed, and if modern radiation therapy techniques are applied.

The results of adjuvant therapy with regard to serum PSA are somewhat controversial. Lange et al.[20] noted that approximately 30% of patients had their PSA fall to the non-detectable region. Link et al.[22] corroborated this early reduction in PSA, but noted that in the majority, the PSA had again begun to rise within a year. More recently, Andriole et al.[21] have reported the use of the 5-alpha reductase inhibitor, finasteride, to delay any subsequent PSA rise in margin-positive patients after radical prostatectomy.

The use of adjuvant hormonal androgen ablation in patients undergoing radical prostatectomy who are seen to have advanced disease is controversial. The group from the Mayo Clinic[23] has demonstrated impressive outcomes in patients with pelvic lymph-node metastasis undergoing radical prostatectomy who receive adjuvant hormonal manipulation. It is unknown whether these patients derived benefit from

Table 9.9 Local recurrence after radical prostatectomy alone

Author	No. Patients	Pathological Stage	Recurrence (%)	Follow-up (Yrs.)
Culp[53]	123	B	26	1–14
Walsh[54]	57	B	12	15
Tomlinson[55]	24	C	8	2–14
Robey[56]	13	C	31	15
Gibbons[6]	51	B + C	10	15
Middleton[57]	22	C	9	5
Catalona[58]	9	C	11	6 Mean
Zincke[59]	47	C,D1	28	4.9 Mean
Catalona[58]	12	D1	25	7.5 Mean
Steinberg[60]	64	D1	11	3.8 Mean

the surgical procedure itself or only from the hormonal manipulation. Further investigation in this arena is certainly necessary before definitive conclusions are possible. Randomized trials evaluating this modality are also underway.

In summary, radical prostatectomy by the retropubic or perineal route is now felt by many to afford the best opportunity for cure in men with localized prostatic carcinoma. Considerable progress has been made towards the reduction of morbidity and this, coupled with an increasing incidence of diagnosis in patients with a more favourable pathological stage, has resulted in considerable enthusiasm for radical prostatectomy. The definitive answer as to whether radical prostatectomy actually results in a reduction in cancer-related mortality awaits the conclusion of three ongoing trials that randomize men to radical prostatectomy versus watchful waiting. A Swedish study is currently enrolling patients. An MRC study has commenced in the United Kingdom. The recently funded Prostate Intervention and Observation Trial (PIVOT) in the US will randomize 2 000 men to radical prostatectomy versus observation, and will use all causes of mortality as the definitive endpoint. In the absence of the definitive answers that these studies will provide, it seems reasonable to offer radical prostatectomy to fitter, younger men with clinically localized prostate cancer and at least a 10-year life expectancy, provided that the patients are carefully counselled about the risks and benefits and have all other options explained to them.

RADIATION THERAPY

Radiation therapy provides an alternative, definitive treatment approach to clinically localized prostatic carcinoma. Radiation therapy has undergone considerable evolution since Paschkis first used cystoscopically applied radium sources to treat prostate cancer. Although various applications of radiation energy were applied to the prostate, followed by cobalt-beam external-radiation therapy, it was the application of the radiation energy derived from linear accelerator by Bagshaw and colleagues at Stanford that changed the course of definitive radiation.

In general, patients being considered for radiation therapy of the prostate should have similar criteria to those undergoing radical prostatectomy (**Table 9.11**). Significant bladder or rectal dysfunction may preclude such treatment approaches.

Problems with pre-operative surgical staging extend to patients being considered for radiation therapy. The issue, however, is intensified somewhat in the radiation therapy series because, in general, definitive

Table 9.10 Adjuvant radiation therapy following radical prostatectomy

Author	Pathological Stage	No.	Local Recurrence (%)	% 5 Years Disease-Free	Follow-up (Years)
Rosenberg[61]	B	34	3	88	3.3 Mean
Gibbons[6]	C	22	5	71	9 Mean
Bahnson[62]	C	14	0	75	5.3 Mean
Rosenberg[61]	C	25	8.0	80	3.3 Mean
Ray[63]	C	13	23	57	5–15
Jacobson[64]	C	26	0	69	5
Lange[65]	C2,C3	35	3	80	4.2 Median
Pilepich[66]	C,D1	18	0	50	3.4 Median
Forman[67]	C,D1	16	0		4 Median
Bahnson[62]	D1	6	17	41	5.3 Median
Rosenberg[61]	D1	12	8	92	3.3 Mean
Lange[65]	D1	36	3	69	4 Median

pelvic-node staging is not provided as these patients rarely undergo lymphadenectomy. Moreover, patients treated with radiation therapy do not have the benefit of having definitive pathological staging.

Table 9.12 illustrates the advantages and disadvantages of this treatment approach. A significant benefit in patients selecting external-beam radiation therapy is the absence of the surgical procedure. The absence of a major operation allows this treatment approach to be added in patients with a less favourable, general medical condition. However, the benefit of treatment of localized prostate cancer and the potential risks must be carefully compared with the patients' overall longevity. Disadvantages of radiation therapy include significant morbidity, including bladder and bowel injury (some patients requiring major surgical intervention for treatment of complications)[24], the time involved with a prolonged treatment course, a high incidence of persistent disease as evidenced by PSA and/or post-radiation positive biopsies, and the potential at least for the development of subsequent primary prostate carcinomas. Furthermore, the anxiety associated with the unknown status of a potentially persistent carcinoma exists in men so treated.

Partial urinary incontinence has been reported to occur in approximately 2% of patients undergoing external-beam radiation therapy, and total urinary incontinence in 1–3% of patients has been reported in large series[25,26,27]. A major potential complication – that of sufficient rectal injury to demand construction of a colostomy – has been reported in up to 3% of patients undergoing external-beam radiation therapy[27].

In properly selected patients, external-beam radiation therapy affords a 15-year overall survival, similar to that observed in patients treated with radical prostatectomy. For example, Hanks[28] compared the survival in 3 series comprised of 134 patients receiving external-beam radiation therapy by the Stanford group[29], with 195 patients treated at Virginia Mason Medical Center[30], and with 57 treated at the Johns Hopkins Medical Center with radical prostatectomy[31]. The 15-year overall survivals were 52%, 57% and 51% respectively. Impressive results have extended to even more advanced cases (clinical stage C, T3–T4). For example, Perez et al.[26] found 5-year NED (no evidence of disease) survival rates of 54%. Zagars et al.[32] noted 15-year disease-free survival rates of 40% in such patients.

Perhaps even more enlightening is the compilation reported by Epstein[33], which is shown in Table 9.13. These series are noteworthy in that all patients underwent staging pelvic lymphadenectomy in conjunction with radical prostatectomy, or prior to external-beam radiation therapy.

Table 9.11 Criteria for radiation therapy
Histological evidence of prostate cancer
Clinically localized disease*
Sufficient life expectancy to render cure worthwhile
Absence of lower urinary-tract disorder
Absence of colorectal disease
Absence of recent or pending TURP
Adequate informed consent
* Some investigators may extend to T3–T4

Table 9.12 Advantages and disadvantages of radiation therapy	
Advantages	Disadvantages
Potential cure	Prolonged treatment (EBRT)
Avoid surgery	Difficulty assessing cure
	Patient anxiety in follow-up
	No definitive staging
	No effect on BPH
	Potential mortality
	Potential morbidity including: rectal injury, bladder damage, incontinence, impotence, haematuria
	May not be necessary

Advances in external-beam radiation therapy have occurred in several arenas, most importantly in the appropriate selection of patients to receive such therapy, similar to the situation for patients undergoing radical prostatectomy. Moreover, recently conformal approaches have resulted in decreasing radiation doses to surrounding tissue, such as the bladder and rectum, with the potential for reduction in morbidity[34,35]. One difficulty in looking at the historical external-beam radiation series is the possibility that relatively inaccurate pelvic imaging techniques used in the determination of the radiation portals may have resulted in significant underdosing or actually missing portions of the prostate[36,37].

Interstitial Radiotherapy

Another approach to the radiation therapy of the prostate is interstitial or brachytherapy. This technique, in which radioactive sources are implanted permanently or temporarily into the prostate, has

undergone considerable evolution, particularly with respect to using imaging modalities (most recently transrectal ultrasound) to afford better distribution of the radiation source. The initial experience employing Iodine-125 has been shown, in long-term follow-up, to have prohibitively high local and metastatic recurrence rates[38]. Improvements in imaging modalities, including both computed tomography for pre-operative evaluation of the prostate anatomy and selection of the implantation pattern, and the use of transrectal ultrasound to guide the surgical procedure itself, may result in a reduction in the failure rate.

Traditionally, Iodine-125 implantations were first performed by open surgical implantation through a retropubic incision[39]. Pelvic lymphadenectomy was performed and thus, in the initial series, accurate pathological staging of the status of the lymph nodes was carried out. Implantation of the radioisotope was performed with an attempt at manually providing uniform spacing of the needles. Dosimetry calculations were carried out pre-operatively. Although many problems intrinsic to this technique led to its eventual abandonment, the biggest problem had to do with inhomogeneity of the seed implantation. This resulted in significant 'underdosing' of areas in the prostate. Indeed, studies using current imaging modalities performed on patients having undergone Iodine-125 implantation by historical techniques demonstrated that this underdosing may have occurred in up to 40% of patients[40].

In addition to improved imaging techniques, expectations of brachytherapy have increased owing to the ability for computerized dose calculations which, in conjunction with topographic templates, allow accurate control of radiation dosing. Significant complications associated with brachytherapy include injury to the bladder and/or rectum. One potential benefit is a decreased incidence of erectile dysfunction relative to external-beam or radical prostatectomy series.

Modern approaches to brachytherapy all use transperineal approaches, which obviates the need for a surgical incision. A perineal template affords control of needle insertion.

One advantage of the newer isotopes is the higher energy afforded by them. The low, prolonged half-life of Iodine-125 was theorized to have some advantage in slow-growing prostatic carcinoma. However, the potential exists that tumour cells with more rapid proliferation rates may repopulate faster than they can be eliminated with the low-dose energy. Paladium-103, with its shorter half-life, delivers a greater hourly dose

Table 9.13 Patterns of failure (%) after radiation therapy or surgery, stage B prostate cancer			
Reference	68*	57**	11
Treatment method	EBRT	RP	RP
Any recurrence			
5-year	15	10	11
10-year	33	50	–
Local recurrence			
5-year	4	7	4
10-year	14	4	–
Cause-specific survival			
5-year	4	3	3
10-year	14	17	–
Survival			
5-year	87	94	93
10-year	63	67	–

EBRT = External-beam radiotherapy
RP = Radical prostatectomy
* Actuarial
** Absolute, lost patients eliminated

than slower-acting Iodine-125. Iridium-192 has a prolonged half-life, but its increased energy (requiring after-loading application) may be advantageous. Long-term follow-up is necessary before claims of actual improvement in cancer-specific mortality and local control with these new isotopes can be assessed. Additionally, several series currently accruing patients combine brachytherapy with external-beam radiation therapy.

OUTCOME AFTER RADIOTHERAPY

The evaluation of patients following radiation therapy of the prostate includes those tests useful for the patients after radical prostatectomy. However, in this setting, PSA is less well characterized, in that detectable serum levels of PSA are usually identified following radiation therapy. While several reports[41-45] have correlated the absence of progression with the nadir of PSA, the definitive identification of the nadir level and the duration of the nadir associated with improved prognosis have not been adequately determined.

One additional approach to the evaluation of patients following radiation therapy of the prostate is the ability to perform prostate needle biopsies. A number of studies have demonstrated considerably high rates of positive biopsies in this setting. For example, Freiha et al. noted that 68% of patients with stage B2 or C prostate cancer have positive biopsies[46]. They correlated the presence of a positive biopsy with clinical recurrence. Similar data have been provided by Scardino et al.[47], who reviewed post-radiation biopsy in 803 men undergoing pelvic lymphadenectomy, radioactive gold-seed implantation, along with external-beam radiation therapy. Of 124 patients who had 1 or more biopsies performed, 6–36 months following completion of radiation therapy 43 (35%) had positive biopsies. These authors demonstrated not only that the incidence of positive biopsy correlated directly with the clinical stage of the tumour, but that local and distant metastases were much more commonly found in those patients with a positive biopsy than those with negative biopsies. This article unequivocally demonstrates the prognostic significance of persistent carcinoma following definitive radiotherapy[47]. Kabalin et al.[48] in a review of 27 men, 18 months or more following radiation therapy, demonstrated positive biopsies in 25 (93%). Of note, 20 of the 22 patients with normal feeling prostates on rectal examination had residual carcinoma. Furthermore, 10 of 12 patients with a serum PSA less than 10.0 ng/ml had positive biopsies, and all men with a PSA greater than this (15) had persistent carcinoma.

In contrast, Kuban et al.[49] noted that only 18% of patients with in general more favourable clinical stage had positive biopsies. One concern in this regard is the often exceedingly difficult diagnostic dilemma that the pathologist is faced with in the determination of post-radiation biopsies. Immunohistochemistry with high molecular weight cytokeratin has been shown to be a helpful adjunct in this regard[50] (see Chapter 2).

It is of course appealing to attempt to compare radical prostatectomy to radiation therapy. Unfortunately, definitive answers are currently impossible owing to the absence of adequately controlled, randomized prospective trials in this regard. An attempt at such a trial by the Intergroup Network in the United States failed owing to poor patient enrollment. One study did randomize patients to radical prostatectomy versus external-beam radiation therapy. Paulson et al. reported on a prospective, randomized trial of men with stage T1–T2 prostate cancer[51]. Unfortunately, this study has been criticized for a number of reasons, including problems associated with the initial randomization, as well as delivery of the assigned treatment. Other methodological problems, including data analysis, have also been raised. This study does, however, remain the only report in which patients were randomized, and demonstrates earlier first evidence of treatment failure in those patients receiving radiation therapy.

Table 9.14 illustrates that local tumour control (which is arguably the best way to compare local treatment) rate for low-stage prostatic carcinoma is approximately equivalent across all treatment modalities, including radical prostatectomy, external-beam radiation therapy and brachytherapy. Obviously, significant differences in patient mix and the absence of randomized trials obviate the ability to adequately compare the efficacy of therapy. It is of note that the efficacy of implantation of radiation appears to fall behind that of external-beam radiation therapy for more advanced disease.

Recently, Stamey et al.[52] reported on 124 consecutive unselected patients who had serial PSA following definitive external-beam radiation therapy. After a follow-up of 32 months, 51% of the patients had increasing values, while 41% were stable. The series was updated with additional follow-up of 48 months on 113 patients, and a mean over follow-up of 6 years. Seventy-eight percent of men had precipitously increasing PSA. In 23 men (20%), stable PSA values of less than 1.7 and a mean follow-up of 9 years were reported; these men were deemed by these authorities to be 'cured'. No correlation between clinical stage and the PSA evidence of progression versus cure was noted.

CONCLUSIONS

The treatment of clinically localized prostatic adenocarcinoma has evolved, and continues to evolve owing to a variety of factors over the past few decades. Men to be considered for such therapy should have at least a 10-year life expectancy, and be made well aware of the controversies surrounding aggressive management as opposed to watchful waiting. Available options for the treatment of such patients include radical prostatectomy, radiation therapy, and more recently cryosurgical ablation of the prostate. Each has significant advantages and disadvantages. The absence of definitive, prospective, randomized trials comparing one mode of therapy to another makes conclusive recommendations for an individual patient impossible. It is therefore encumbent upon the clinician involved in counselling men with localized prostate cancer to most carefully assess the risk:benefit ratio for the individual patient in order to help him and his family decide upon the most appropriate therapeutic option.

Table 9.14 Local tumour control following implantation versus external-beam radiation therapy (EBRT) versus prostatectomy

Treatment	Stage A	Stage B	Stage C	Follow-Up (Years)	Reference
Implant	91% (11)*	74% (32)	56% (32)	3–12	Kuban[69]
	88% (41)		86% (57)	3–7	Kim[70]
	100% (20)			2+	Giles[71]
	100% [a]	83%	71%	3–13	Morton[72]
	100% (3)	95% (38)	85% (13)	2–9	Delaney[73]
	100% (6)	91% (69)	95% (19)	7–13	Reddy[74]
		68% (191)[b]	24% (87)	10	Fuks[75]
		41% (324)[c]		10	Fuks[75]
EBRT	97% (35)	87% (104)	74% (107)	3–12	Kuban[69]
	93% (23)	62% (87)	63% (111)	10	Amdur[25]
	88% (41)	83% (185)	72% (328)	3–16	Perez[26]
	100% (9)	94% (78)	82% (20)	3–13	Morton[72]
Surgery	80% (5)	90% (41)	25% (4)	5	Schellhammer[76]
		90% (52)		15–32	Gibbons[77]
		73% (123)		1–15	Culp[53]

* = Numbers in parentheses represent the number of patients treated
[a] = 141 total patients implanted in series. 18% excluded as 'inadequately treated'. Stage breakdown not provided
[b] = Stage B1 (unilobar, < 2 cm)
[c] = Stage B2 (unilobar, > 2 cm)
Reproduced from K. Wallner[78] with permission

REFERENCES

1. Lange P, Narayan P. Understaging and undergrading of prostate cancer: argument for postoperative radiation as adjuvant therapy. *Urology* 1983;**21**:113–118.

2. Boxer R, Kaufman J, Goodwin W. Radical prostatectomy for carcinoma of the prostate: 1951-1976. A review of 329 patients. *J Urol* 1977;**117**:208213.

3. Catalona W, Stein A. Staging errors in clinically localized prostatic cancer. *J Urol* 1982;**127**:452–456.

4. Veenema R, Gursel E, Lattimer J. Radical retropubic prostatectomy for cancer: a 20-year experience. *J Urol.* 1977;**117**:330–331.

5. Jewett H. The case for radical perineal prostatectomy. *J Urol* 1970;**103**:195–199.

6. Gibbons R, Cole B, Richardson R, *et al.* Adjuvant radiotherapy following radical prostatectomy: Results and complications. *J Urol* 1986;**135**:65–68.

7. Elder J, Jewett J, Walsh P. Radical perineal prostatectomy for clinical stage B2 carcinoma of the prostate. *J Urol* 1982;**127**:704–706.

8. Partin A, Carter H, Chan D, *et al.* Prostate specific antigen in the staging of localized prostate cancer: Influence of tumor differentiation, tumor volume and benign hyperplasia. *J. Urol.* 1990;**143**:747–752.

9. Denis LJ, Murphy GP, Schroder FH. Report of the consensus workshop on screening and global strategy for prostate cancer. *Cancer* 1995;**75**(in press).

10. Reiner W, Walsh P. An anatomical approach to the surgical management to the dorsal vein and Santorini's plexus during radical retropubic surgery. *J Urol.* 1979;**121**:198–200.

11. Walsh PC. Radical retropubic prostatectomy with reduced morbidity: An anatomic approach. *NCI Monogr.* 1988;**7**:133–137.

12. Lepor H, Gregerman M, Crosby R, *et al.* Precise localization of the autonomic nerves from the pelvic plexus to the corpora cavernosa: A detailed anatomical study of the adult male pelvis. *J Urol.* 1985;**133**:207–212.

13. Walsh PC, Donker PJ. Impotence following radical prostatectomy: insight into etiology and prevention. *J Urol.* 1982;**128**:492–497.

14. Quinlan D, Epstein J, Carter B, *et al.* Sexual function following radical prostatectomy: influence of preservation of neurovascular bundles. *J. Urol.* 1991;**145**:998–1002.

15. Catalona W, Basler J. Return of erections and urinary continence following radical retropubic prostatectomy. *J. Urol.* 1993;**150**:905–907.

16. Lu-Yao GL, McLerran D, Wasson J, *et al.* An assessment of radical prostatectomy. *JAMA.* 1993;**269**:2633–2636.

17. Herr HW. Quality of life of incontinent men after radical prostatectomy. *J Urol.* 1994;**151**:652–654.

18. Levy DA, Resnick, M. I. Laparoscopic pelvic lymphadenectomy and radical perineal prostatectomy: A viable alternative to radical retropubic prostatectomy. *J Urol.* 1994;**151**:905–908.

19. Labrie F, Dupont A, Cusan L, *et al.* Downstaging of localized prostate cancer by neoadjuvant therapy with Flutamide and Lupron: the first controlled and randomized trial. *Clin Invest Med.* 1993;**16**:499–509.

20. Lange PH, Lightner DJ, Medini E, *et al.* The effect of radiation therapy after radical prostatectomy in patients with elevated PSA levels. *J Urol.* 1990;**144**:927–932.

21. Andriole GL. Finasteride induced PSA reduction in patients with early stage prostate cancer. *J Urol* 1994;**151(Suppl)**:450A.

22. Link P, Freiha F, Stamey T. Adjuvant radiation therapy in patients with detectable prostate specific antigen following radical prostatectomy. *J Urol* 1991;**145**:532–534.

23. Zincke H. Extended experience with surgical treatment of stage D1 adenocarcinoma of prostate. Significant influence of immediate adjuvant hormonal treatment (orchiectomy) on outcome. *Urology (Suppl).* 1993;**33**:27–36.

24. Hanks GE. Radical prostatectomy or radiation therapy for early prostate cancer: Two roads to the same end. *Cancer.* 1988;**61**:2153–2160.

25. Amdur RJ, Parsons JT, Fitzgerald LT, Million RR. Adenocarcinoma of the prostate treated with external-beam radiation therapy: 5-year minimum follow-up. *Radiother Oncol.* 1990;**18**:235–246.

26. Perez C, Pilepich M, Garcia D, *et al.* Definitive radiation therapy in carcinoma of the prostate localized to the pelvis: experience at the Mallinckrodt Institute of Radiology. *NCI Monogr.* 1988;**7**:85–94.

27. Schellhammer PF, El-Mahdi AM. Pelvic complications after definitive treatment of prostate cancer by interstitial or external beam radiation. *Urology.* 1983;**21**:451–457.

28. Hanks G. Radiotherapy or surgery for prostate cancer: ten and fifteen year results of external beam therapy. *Acta. Oncol.* 1991;**30(2)**:231–237.

29. Bagshaw M, Cox R, Ray G. Status of radiation treatment of prostate cancer. *NCI Monogr.* 1988;**7**:47–60.

30. Gibbons R, Correa R Jr, Brannen,G, *et al.* Total prostatectomy for clinically localized prostatic cancer: Long-term results. *J Urol.* 1989;**131**:564–566.

31. Jewett H, Bridge R, Gray G, *et al.* The palpable nodule prostatic cancer: Results 15 years after radical excision. *JAMA.* 1968;**203**:403–406.

32. Zagars GK, von Eschenbach AC, Johnson DE, *et al.* Stage C adenocarcinoma of the prostate: An analysis of 551 patients treated with external beam radiation. *Cancer.* 1987;**60**:1489–1499.

33. Epstein BE, Hanks GE. Prostate Cancer: Evaluation and Radiotherapeutic Management. *Ca-Cancer J Clin.* 1992;**42**:223–240.

34. Soffen EM, Hanks GE, Hwang CC, *et al.* Conformal static field therapy for low volume low grade prostate cancer with rigid immobilization. *Int J Radiat Oncol Biol Phys.* 1991;**20**:141–146.

35. Soffen EM, Hanks GE, Hunt MA, *et al.* Conformal static field radiation therapy for treatment of early prostate cancer versus non-conformal techniques: A reduction in acute morbidity. *Int J Radiat Oncol Biol Phys.* 1992;**24(3)**:485–488.

36. Asbell SO, Schlager BA, Baker AS. Revision of treatment planning for carcinoma of the prostate. *Int J Radiat Oncol Biol Phys.* 1980;**6**:861–865.

37. Lee DJ, Leibel S, Shiels R, *et al.* The value of ultrasonic imaging and CT scanning in planning the radiotherapy for prostatic carcinoma. *Cancer.* 1980;**45**:724–727.

38. Wallner K, Chie-Tsao ST, Roy J et al. An improved method for computerized tomography-planned transperineal 125 iodine prostate implants. J Urol. 1991;**146**:90–95.

39. Whitmore W Jr, Hilaris B, Grabstald H. Retropubic implantation of iodine-125 in the treatment of prostatic cancer. J Urol 1972;**108**:918–920.

40. Stone NN, Forman JD, Sogani PC, et al. Transrectal ultrasonography and I-125 implantation in patients with prostate cancer. J Urol. 1988;**139**:604A.

41. Zagars GK, von Eschenbach AC. PSA: an important marker for prostate cancer treated by external beam therapy. Cancer. 1993;**72**:538–548.

42. Zietman AL Coen JJ, Shipley WU, et al.. Adjuvant irradiation after radical prostatectomy for adenocarcinoma of prostate: analysis of freedom from PSA failure. Urology. 1993;**42**: 292–299.

43. Kaplan ID, Cox RS, Bagshaw MA. Prostate Specific Antigen after External Beam Radiotherapy for Prostatic Cancer: Follow-up. J Urol. 1993;**149**:519–522.

44. Schellhammer P, El-Mahdi A, Wright G, et al. Prostate-specific antigen to determine progression-free survival after radiation therapy for localized carcinoma of prostate. J Urol. 1993;**42**:13–20.

45. Zietman AL, Coen JJ, Shipley WU, et al. Radical radiation therapy in the management of prostatic adenocarcinoma: the initial prostate specific antigen value as a predictor of treatment outcome. J Urol. 1994;**151**:640–645.

46. Freiha F, Bagshaw M. Carcinoma of the prostate: Results of post-irradiation biopsy. Prostate. 1984;**5(1)**:19–25.

47. Scardino PT, Frankel JM, Wheeler TM, et al. The prognostic significance of postirradiation biopsy results in patients with prostatic cancer. J. Urol. 1986;**135(3)**:510–516.

48. Kabalin J, Hodge K, McNeal J, et al.. Identification of residual cancer in the prostate following radiation therapy: Role of transrectal ultrasound guided biopsy and prostate specific antigen. J Urol. 1989;**142**:326–331.

49. Kuban DA, el-Mahdi AM, Schellhammer PF, et al. The significance of post-irradiation biopsy with long-term follow-up. Int J Radiat Oncol Biol Phys. 1992;**24(3)**:409–414.

50. Brawer M, Nagle R, Pitts W et al. Keratin immunoreactivity as an aid to the diagnosis of persistent adenocarcinoma in irradiated human prostates. Cancer. 1989;**63(3)**:454–460.

51. Paulson D, Lin G, Hinshaw W, et al. Radical surgery versus radiotherapy for adenocarcinoma of the prostate. J Urol. 1982;**128(3)**: 502–504.

52. Stamey T, Ferrari, M, Schmid H. Value of serial prostate specific antigen determinations 5 years after radiotherapy: steeply increasing values characterize 80% of patients. J. Urol. 1993;**150**:1845–1850.

53. Culp OS. Radical perineal prostatectomy: its past, present, and possible future. J Urol. 1968;**98**:618–626.

54. Walsh P, Jewett H. Radical surgery for prostatic cancer. Cancer. 1980;**45**:1906–1911.

55. Tomlinson R, Currie D, Boyce W. Radical prostatectomy: palliation for stage C carcinoma of the prostate. J Urol. 1977;**117(1)**:85–87.

56. Robey E, Schellhammer P. Local failure after definitive therapy for prostatic cancer. J Urol. 1987; **137(4)**:613–619.

57. Middleton R, Smith J Jr, Melzer R, et al. Patient survival and local recurrence rate following radical prostatectomy for prostatic carcinoma. J Urol. 1986;**136**:422–424.

58. Catalona W, Miller D, Kavoussi L. Intermediate-term survival results in clinically understaged prostate cancer patients following radical prostatectomy. J Urol 1988;**142(3)**: 832–833.

59. Zincke H, Utz DC, Taylor WF. Bilateral pelvic lymphadenectomy and radical prostatectomy for clinical stage C prostatic cancer: role of adjuvant treatment for residual cancer and in disease progression. J Urol. 1986;**135**: 1199–1205.

60. Steinberg G, Epstein J, Piantados S, et al.. Management of Stage D1 adenocarcinoma of the prostate: the Johns Hopkins experience 1974–1987. J Urol. 1989;**141**: 310A.

61. Rosenberg S, Loening S, Hawtrey C, et al. Radical prostatectomy with adjuvant radioactive gold for prostatic cancer: a preliminary report. J Urol. 1985;**133(2)**:225–227.

62. Bahnson R, Garnett J, Grayhack J. Adjuvant radiation therapy in stages C and D1 prostatic adenocarcinoma: preliminary results. Urology. 1986; **27(5)**:403–406.

63. Ray G, Bagshaw M, Freiha F. External beam radiation salvage for residual or recurrent local tumor following radical prostatectomy. J Urol. 1984;**132(5)**:926–930.

64. Jacobson G, Simith J Jr, Stewart J. Postoperative radiation therapy for pathologic stage C prostate cancer. Int J Radiat Oncol Biol Phys. 1987;**13(7)**:1021–1024.

65. Lange P, Reddy P, Medini E, et al. Radiation therapy as adjuvant treatment after radical prostatectomy. NCI Monogr. 1988;**7**:141–149.

66. Pilepich M, Walz B, Baglan R. Postoperative irradiation in carcinoma of the prostate. Int J Radiat Oncol Biol Phys. 1984;**10(10)**:1869–1873.

67. Forman J, Wharam M, Lee D, et al. Definitive radiotherapy following prostatectomy: Results and complications. Int J Radiat Oncol Biol Phys. 1986;**12**:185–189.

68. Hanks GE, Asbell S, Krall JM, et al. Outcome for lymph node dissection negative T-1b, T-2 (A-2,B) prostate cancer treated with external beam radiation therapy in RTOG 77-06. Int J Radiat Oncol Biol Phys. 1991;**21**:1099–1103.

69. Kuban DA, El-Mahdi AM, Schellhammer PF. Interstitial implantation for prostate cancer. What have we learned 10 years later? Cancer. 1989;**63**:2415–2420.

70. Kim RY, Bueschen AJ. Interstitial iodine-125 seed implantation in the management of prostate cancer: preliminary report at UAB. Ala Med. 1986;**55(7)**:27–33.

71. Giles GM, Brady LW. Iodine implantation after lymphadenectomy in early carcinoma of the prostate. Int J Radiat Oncol Biol Phys. 1986;**12**:2117–2125.

72. Morton JD, Peschel RE. Iodine-125 implants versus external beam therapy for stages A2, B and C prostate cancer. Int J Radiat Oncol Biol Phys. 1988;**14**:1153–1157.

73. DeLaney TF, Shipley WU, O'Leary MP, et al. Preoperative irradiation, lymphadenectomy, and 125 iodine implantation for patients with localized carcinoma of the prostate. Int J Radiat Oncol Biol Phys. 1986;**12**:1779–1785.

74. Reddy EK, Mebust WK, Weigel JW. Iodine 125 implantation in localized prostatic cancer. Endocuriether Hypertherm Oncol. 1990;**6**:239–244.

75. Fuks Z, Leibel SA, Wallner KE, et al. The effect of local control on metastatic dissemination in carcinoma of the prostate: long-term results in patients treated with 125I implantation. Int J Radiat Oncol Biol Phys. 1991;**21**:537–547.

76. Schellhammer PF. Radical prostatectomy; Patterns of local failure and survival in 67 patients. *Urology*. 1988;**31**:191–197.

77. Gibbons R, Correa R Jr, Brannen G, *et al*. Total prostatectomy for localized prostatic cancer. *J Urol*. 1984;**131(1)**:73–76.

78. Wallner K. Iodine 125 Brachytherapy for early stage prostate cancer: New techniques may achieve better results. *Oncology*. 1991;**5**:115–122.

79. Weldon VE. Radical Perineal Prostatectomy. In Das S, Crawford ED (eds.) *Cancer of the Prostate*. New York: Marcel Dekker, 1993:225–266.

CHAPTER 10

ALTERNATIVE STRATEGIES FOR LOCALIZED PROSTATE CANCER

INTRODUCTION

Although the standard management of localized prostate cancer (at least in younger men) has usually been either radical prostatectomy or external beam radiotherapy, a number of publications have highlighted the fact that a policy of 'watchful waiting' and the deferral of therapy until symptoms arise may be appropriate in smaller volume, well-differentiated lesions, especially in patients with a life expectancy of less than 10 years[1-3]. The difficulties with a policy of watchful waiting include, of course, the anxieties shared by both the patient and urologist that the tumour may advance silently to an incurable stage before definitive therapy is initiated. For this reason there has been a move by some towards alternative strategies to deal with localized prostatic cancer that do not involve the small (but significant) morbidity associated with standard therapies discussed in the previous chapter. It has to be pointed out that however attractive these new more conservative treatment strategies may be, there are as yet no long-term outcome data to inform us about their safety and efficacy. Accordingly, all of them, with the exception of watchful waiting, should be regarded as investigational at present.

WATCHFUL WAITING

Although the concept of watchful waiting often seems difficult to countenance in the presence of proven malignant disease, there is now mounting evidence that in certain patients with prostate cancer this may well be the appropriate course of action. In T1a cancers, diagnosed incidentally at transurethral resection of the prostate for obstructive symptoms, for example, the probability of disease progression over 8 years has been reported to be as low as 3%[4] in one series, and 16% in another[5]. Certainly, in patients with a life expectancy of less than 10 years, most clinicians would adopt a 'wait and see' policy with regular PSA monitoring, proceeding to therapy only if there were clear evidence of disease progression.

Even in patients with more significant volumes of localized prostate cancer present, long-term follow-up studies have suggested a relatively low metastatic rate[3,6]. Although most patients exhibited local disease progression, the majority died of intercurrent diseases rather than prostatic cancer[3].

In a recent meta-analysis of conservative treatment of non-metastatic prostate cancer, Chodak et al.[2] concluded that histological grading provided the best indicator of the probability of significant disease progression. Those patients with grade 1, well-differentiated lesions had a low metastatic rate and an excellent disease-specific survival of 87% at 10 years. By contrast, only 26% of individuals with grade 3, poorly differentiated tumours were still alive 10 years after diagnosis.

Using a decision-analysis mathematical model, Fleming et al.[7] have calculated that conservative therapy may well be the best option for men with well-differentiated, localized prostate cancer, whose life expectancy does not exceed 10 years. However, this study focused on potent men over the age of 60 – those most likely to have side-effects from treatment – and used a rather simplified model of the natural history of prostate cancer. In addition, the data used to predict outcome of treatment did not reflect the results attainable with modern methods of detection and treatment.

CRYOABLATION

Cryoablation – that is, the use of freezing techniques to destroy prostatic tissue, was first utilized by Gonder et al. in 1964[8]. The original concept was that this form of therapy could permanently eliminate all primary tumour in the prostate, while preserving functional and structural integrity of surrounding structures, including the neurovascular bundles. In addition, it was hoped that cryosurgery might induce some form of protective immune response within the host[9]; however, there has never been any scientific evidence to support this concept.

Current techniques of cryoablation employ newly developed technology. The patient is anaesthetized and placed in the lithotomy position. The perineum is prepared and draped, and a suprapubic catheter inserted percutaneously. Urethral warming is accomplished by circulating heated water (at 44 °C) through a urethral catheter. Real-time transrectal ultrasound is then performed to determine the prostatic dimensions. An 18-gauge needle is placed into the prostate and a J-shaped guide wire placed through the needle, deep into the prostatic substance. The track is then dilated and a 7 mm cryoprobe inserted. Three to eight cryoprobes may be inserted in this manner and transrectal ultrasound is employed to monitor correct probe placement (**10.1**). Next, liquid nitrogen is passed into the probes and the freezing process is observed on transrectal ultrasound; as the so-called 'ice balls' develop, their location can be visualized on transrectal ultrasound as they advance through the prostatic tissue to include the prostatic capsule, but they must stop short of the rectal wall. Each of the cryoprobe tips achieves a temperature of between −180°C and −190°C, and produces tissue destruction by inducing intracellular ice crystals which cause cell membrane rupture and protein denaturation in the frozen zone.

While Gonder[8] originally utilized transurethral cryosurgery, which of course limited his ability to treat the peripheral zone of the prostate, Flocks[10], in 1969, used an open perineal exposure for controlled application of cryotherapy under direct vision. Rather later, Bonney and associates[11] used a similar open transperineal approach with visual monitoring of prostate freezing in 229 patients. At five-year follow-up, they noticed a stage-survival probability equivalent to that of radical prostatectomy, but reported an incidence of urethro-rectal fistula of 1.4%, urethro-cutaneous fistula rate of 10.7%, and erectile dysfunction in 7.4% of patients. In a subsequent publication, Bonney[12] reported that although 66% of patients had elimination of palpable tumour, at least 41% suffered recurrent disease and more than 50% of patients received concomitant endocrine therapy. The addition of this adjuvant therapy, unfortunately, confounds attempts to evaluate the true efficacy of this particular modality. More recently, Onik and associates[13] have reported the use of transrectal ultrasound-guided percutaneous transperineal cryosurgery on the prostate of 6 dogs. They reported that with this technique they were able to complete the freezing process successfully and avoid any injury to the rectum and urethra. Following this work, their preliminary results on 55 patients were published. The report was too early to provide reliable information about the efficiency of tumour ablation. However, complications were noted; in particular, four patients suffered freezing of the rectum, leading to urethro-rectal fistula in two and sloughing of prostatic urethral tissue in three. In addition, 65% of patients

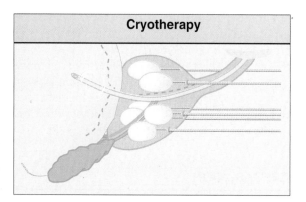

10.1 Cryotherapy: under ultrasound control, up to 8 cryoprobes are introduced into the prostate by the transperineal route. Freezing is accomplished by circulation of liquid nitrogen through the needles while the urethra is protected by warming through a catheter.

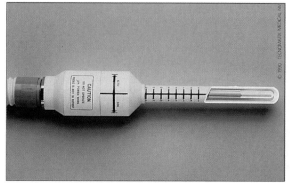

10.2 A transrectal microwave probe for hyperthermia treatment of the prostate.

who were potent pre-therapy were impotent following treatment, indicating probable involvement of the neurovascular bundles in the freezing process.

In the final analysis, the safety and efficacy of cryosurgery for prostatic cancer can only be evaluated by careful long-term follow-up of large numbers of patients, ideally in a long-term randomized study comparing it against standard treatment therapies. At the time of writing, no such data are available.

HYPERTHERMIA TREATMENT

Hyperthermia has for many years been recognized as inducing destruction of various tissues, and it has been suggested that it has a selective cytotoxic effect on tumour cells both *in vitro* and *in vivo*. Although the explanation for this is not entirely clear, it has been proposed that abnormal tumour vessels are incapable of dilating in the presence of heat (as normal vessels are able to do) and that this may render the tumour more susceptible to heat damage. In addition, neoplastic cells appear in some way intrinsically more sensitive to heat than normal cells. The prostate is easily accessible for hyperthermia via the transrectal route (**10.2**).

Investigations into the clinical effects of hyperthermia on neoplastic prostate tissue have so far been limited. Yerushalmi and co-workers were the first to report the use of microwave hypothermia delivered transrectally for local or locally advanced prostate cancer[14]. In their small series of 15 patients, ten were stage C, one was stage B and four were stage D. All but one had severe local symptoms and each was given at least six treatments, lasting an average of one hour, at temperatures of between 42°C and 43°C. Each patient was treated on an out-patient basis without anaesthesia. Unfortunately, some patients were also given adjunctive post-treatment radiotherapy and some were also treated with either oral oestrogens or orchiectomy prior to hyperthermia treatment. Marked improvements in symptoms were reported in all patients. Minimal complications were described, although follow-up was rather short. The same author followed this report in 1986 with a further report of 32 patients similarly treated, again with sporadic employment of adjunctive radiation or hormonal therapy[15]. In this report, the few patients treated with hyperthermia alone appeared to have objective tumour regression, but there was usually evidence of relapse after six months. The best results seemed to be obtained in the 20 patients who were treated with both combined radiotherapy and hyperthermia. Montorsi *et al.*[16] reported the results in 46 patients with locally extensive prostatic cancer presenting with urinary retention or perineal pain in spite of total androgen blockade. Hyperthermia was delivered transrectally in ten one-hour sessions delivered over five weeks, with a calculated intraprostatic temperature of around 43.5°C. This group reported significant improvement of obstructive symptoms and 50% of patients who were in urinary retention were rendered free of their catheter with only minimal complications.

More recently, Servadio and Leib reported a series of 44 patients treated with transrectal hyperthermia in combination with either radiotherapy or hormonal therapy[17]. Twenty-seven of these patients had locally advanced disease, and all had severe local obstruction and irritative symptoms of urinary retention. They noted no complications attributable to hyperthermia, and a significant subjective improvement of symptoms was reported in the majority of patients. Only two of the 27 patients had progression of the disease at four-year follow-up, and nine of the 11 patients who underwent follow-up biopsy were reported to have negative biopsy results. Most recently, Sorensen[18] reported 12 patients undergoing transurethral microwave thermotherapy using the Prostatron™ microwave thermotherapy device (**10.3**). All patients underwent radical prostatectomy 6–9 days after microwave treatment. The depth of the effective injury was 1–1.5 cm, with a well-demarcated line of thermal damage. Tumours situated posteriorly in the peripheral zone, which constitute the majority of prostate cancers, appeared unaffected by this treatment.

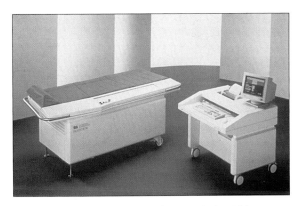

10.3 The Prostatron™ thermotherapy device. This machine delivers microwave energy transurethrally to the prostate while the urethra is cooled by fluid circulated through the urethral catheter.

From these data it seems clear that microwave hyperthermia as a treatment for localized prostate cancer is currently only at an early stage of development. Unfortunately, its true efficacy is difficult to judge from those studies that have been performed, either because no clear protocol was followed, or because adjunctive therapies were employed as well as hyperthermia. None the less, the technique does seem to hold some promise, and hopefully more properly controlled longer-term data will be available in the future.

LASER THERAPY

Laser treatment of localized prostate cancer has also been investigated. Lasers transform light energy into heat within the prostatic tissue, resulting in an intraprostatic temperature considerably above 60°C for a few seconds. At this temperature, rapid protein denaturation and cell necrosis result. The depth of penetration of light (and therefore the volume of affected tissue) is primarily dependent upon the wave-length of the applied laser light. The recent advent of right-angled laser fibres has allowed more precise application of the laser energy to the prostate (**10.4**).

Sander and Beisland[19] pioneered the use of the neodymium yag (Nd:YAG) laser for the treatment of localized prostate cancer. Nd:YAG laser radiation seemed to produce a homogeneous coagulation to a depth of 3–4 mm without the necessity to remove tissue. The necrotic zone that was created gradually converted into fibrotic scar tissue, with only minor shrinkage. Between 1981 and 1986, over 100 patients with localized lesions were treated with either transurethral or suprapubic access to the gland. A suprapubic trocar for cystoscopy was utilized to access all of the capsular areas of the prostate that were not treatable with the laser fibre transurethrally. All patients initially underwent extended transurethral resection of the prostate, exposing capsular fibres throughout the extent of the resection. Three to five weeks later, a thorough lasering of the prostatic capsular bed was performed using 40–50 watts of laser power applied in bursts of 1–4 seconds; a total of 7 000–21 000 joules were applied. The transformation of tissue into a grey-white mass (checked by visual inspection) was used as an end point for adequate treatment in a given area of the prostate. At a two-year follow-up, 56 of the original 63 patients were deemed disease free, and only 7 cases were regarded as treatment failures. The failures occurred in patients in whom only the transurethral approach was used.

Samdal and Brevick[20] reported rather similar results in 26 patients with localized prostate cancer: all patients underwent extended TURP followed in 6 weeks by Nd:YAG laser treatment at 45 W with a total of 11 000–35 000 J being applied. They reported minimal perioperative complications, but did describe eight late complications: four patients developed bladder neck contracture, two developed stress urinary incontinence, and one developed erectile dysfunction. A further individual developed urethral stenosis and one bilateral hydronephrosis secondary to fibrosis of the ureteric orifices. These authors stressed the importance of careful monitoring of rectal temperature to prevent development of prostato-rectal fistulae. At a rather short follow-up period, 22 of the 26 patients were reported to be disease free. At follow-up, most patients had a reduction in PSA levels, but in no patient did the PSA decrease to undetectable levels.

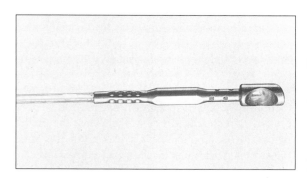

10.4 A side-firing laser probe which may be used to treat the prostate through a cystoscope (Bard Urolase[R]).

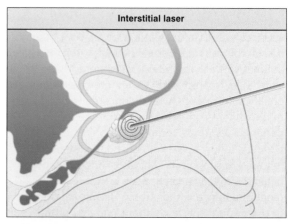

10.5 Interstitial laser therapy of the prostate involves the transperineal placement of a laser fibre into the prostate. Laser energy is converted into thermal energy within the gland, resulting in localized tissue destruction.

Lately, interest has been increasing in the use of interstitial laser therapy for prostate cancer, using percutaneous placement of the needles in order to deliver Nd:YAG laser energy (**10.5**). Littrup and associates[21] reported a study in dogs demonstrating focal intraprostatic areas of necrosis and coagulation extending up to 14 mm. Although needles could be placed accurately using ultrasound, the extent of laser treatment was rather imprecise, as the penetration depth of tissue damage was variable.

Other means of delivering laser energy to the prostate are currently being investigated. Liong and colleagues[22] have reported the use of a transurethral balloon 'laserthermia' device that emits circumferential laser energy. Initial studies in dogs revealed extensive coagulation necrosis of the prostatic tissue together with subsequent cavitation formation. Early studies in men with BPH have been encouraging, but clearly this device also carries possibilities for the treatment of patients with localized prostate cancer. As yet, however, no data are available concerning its efficacy for this application.

HIGH INTENSITY FOCUSED ULTRASOUND

Technological advances in extracorporeal therapy have produced high intensity focused ultrasound (HIFU) as a new modality for the management of prostatic diseases. The transrectal route is employed, which allows real-time ultrasound imaging of the intraprostatic lesions created. The technique depends upon the creation of foci of cytotoxic intraprostatic temperatures at the points of convergence of the ultrasound beams. The temperatures at these points may exceed 100°C (**10.6**).

High intensity focused ultrasound

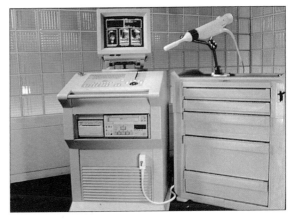

b) The HIFU machine.

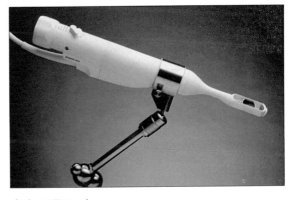

10.6 High intensity focused ultrasound (HIFU) energy may be delivered to the prostate transrectally. At the point of intersection of ultrasound waves extremely high temperatures are delivered, resulting in tissue destruction.
a) Diagrammatic representation.

c) The HIFU probe.

As yet, the results of treatment of only canine prostate (**10.7**) and benign prostatic hyperplasia in men (**10.8**) have been reported[23,24], but phase II studies of patients with localized prostate cancer are now underway. Their results in terms of effective PSA suppression and subsequent biopsy data are awaited with considerable interest.

ADJUVANT ANDROGEN DEPRIVATION

The recent publication of so many reports suggesting benefit from combining androgen deprivation with other local therapies directed at the prostate tumour itself, probably reflects the fact that no currently available therapy for localized prostate cancer is completely effective[25, 26]. As described in Chapter 9, neoadjuvant therapy with LHRH analogues before either radical prostatectomy[27] or conformed radiotherapy[28] has been reported as improving the results of treatment. It seems likely that in the future antiandrogens such as Casodex or flutamide will be used in combination with local therapies such as cryosurgery[29] or HIFU. Such combinations are currently under investigation. The real benefits in terms of freedom from progression and overall survival of such combination therapies will need to be carefully evaluated by long-term randomized studies.

CONCLUSIONS

Watchful waiting with deferred introduction of endocrine ablation when symptoms develop is now a legitimate treatment option for patients with low-volume, well-differentiated prostate cancer and/or limited life expectancy. There has been a recent, rapid development of new, minimally invasive technologies for dealing with bladder-outflow obstruction due to BPH. It seems likely that a similar trend may be seen in prostatic cancer. Of course, this problem is an intrinsically more difficult one in that urologists will wish to be confident that all cancer tissue has been reliably ablated by new competitor therapies to radical prostatectomy and external-beam radiotherapy. To date, there is no conclusive evidence to suggest that any of the new technologies available thus far is capable of producing long-term tumour ablation with reliable serum PSA suppression and minimal side-effects. However, there is little doubt that there is potential for further developments in this area.

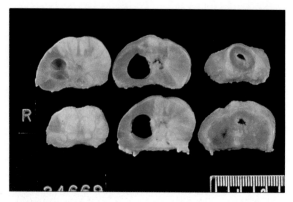

10.7 Lesions in the dog prostate created by the HIFU device.

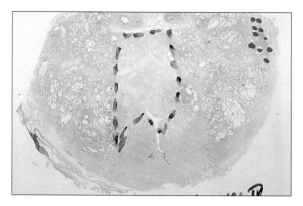

10.8 Lesion created in prostate of patient with BPH with HIFU device.

REFERENCES

1 Adolfsson J. Deferred treatment of low grade stage T3 prostate cancer without distant metastases. J Urol 1993; **149**:326–329.

2 Chodak GW, Thisted RA, Gerber GS, *et al*. Results of conservative management of clinically localized prostate cancer. *New Eng J Med* 1994;**4**:242–248.

3 George NJR. Natural history of localised prostatic cancer managed by conservative therapy alone. *Lancet* 1988;494–497.

4 Cantrell BB, DeKlerk DP, Eggleston JC, *et al*. Pathological factors that influence prognosis in stage A prostatic cancer: the influence of extent versus grade. J Urol 1981;**125**:516–521.

5 Epstein JI, Paull G, Eggleston JC, *et al*. Prognosis of untreated stage A1 prostatic carcinoma: a study of 94 cases with extended follow-up. J Urol 1986;**136**:837–839.

6 Johansson JE, Adami HO, Andersson SO, *et al*. High 10-year survival rate in patients with early, untreated prostatic cancer. JAMA 1992;**267**:2191–2196.

7 Fleming C, Wasson JH, Albertsen PC, *et al*. A decision analysis of alternate treatment strategies for clinically localized prostate cancer. JAMA 1993;269:2650–2658.

8 Gonder MH, Soanes WA, Smith V. Experimental prostate cryosurgery. *Invest Urol* 1964;**1**:610–618.

9 Soanes WA, Ablin RJ, Gonder MJ. Remission of metastatic lesions following cryosurgery in prostate cancer. J Urol 1970;**104**:154–159.

10 Flocks TH, Nelson CMK, Boatman CL. Perineal cryosurgery for prostatic carcinoma. J Urol 1972;**108**:933–935.

11 Bonney WW, Platz CE, Fallon B, *et al*. Cryosurgery in prostatic cancer: survival. *Urology* 1982;**19**:37–42.

12 Bonney WW, Fallen B, Gerber WL, *et al*. Cryosurgery in prostatic cancer: elimination of the local lesion. *Urology* 1983;**22**:8–15.

13 Onik GM, Cohen JK, Reyes GD, *et al*. Transrectal ultrasound-guided percutaneous radical cryosurgical ablation of the prostate. *Cancer* 1993;**72(4)**:1291–1299.

14 Yerushalmi A, Servadio C, Leib C, *et al*. Local hyperthermia for treatment of carcinoma of the prostate: a preliminary report. *Prostate* 1982;**3**:623–629.

15 Yerushalmi A, Shani A, Fishelovitz Y, *et al*. Local microwave hyperthermia in the treatment of carcinoma of the prostate. *Oncology* 1986;**43**:299–305.

16 Montorsi F, Guazzoni G, Colombo R, *et al*. Transrectal microwave hyperthermia for advanced prostate cancer: long-term clinical results. J Urol 1992;**148**:342–345.

17 Servadio C, Leib Z. Local hyperthermia for prostate cancer. *Urology* 1991;**38**:342–345.

18 Sorensen RB, McGarragle MP, Grignon DJ, *et al*. Transurethral microwave thermotherapy (TUMT) using the Prostatron: a histopathological evaluation of the thermal effects on carcinoma of the prostate. J Urol 1993;**149**:232A.

19 Sander S, Beisland HO. Laser in the treatment of localized prostatic cancer. J Urol 1984;**132**:280–281.

20 Samdal F, Brevik B. Laser combined with TURP in the treatment of localized prostatic cancer. *Scand J Urol Nephrol* 1990;**24**:175–181.

21 Littrup PJ, Lee F, Borlaza GS, *et al*. Percutaneous ablation of canine prostate using transrectal ultrasound guidance absolute ethanol and Nd:YAG laser. *Invest Radiol* 1988;**23**:734–739.

22 Liong ML, Suzuki T, Yamanaka H, *et al*. Prostalase: Basic clinical research and preliminary clinical results with laser thermotherapy for symptomatic benign prostatic hyperplasia. J *Clinic Laser Med & Surg* 1994;**12(2)**:85–92.

23 Bihrle R, Foster RS, Sanghvi NT, *et al*. High intensity focused ultrasound for the treatment of benign prostatic hyperplasia: early United States experience. J Urol 1994;**151**:1271–1275.

24 Madersbacher M, Kratzik C, Szabo N, *et al*. Tissue ablation in benign prostatic hyperplasia with high intensity focused ultrasound. *Eur Urol* 1993;**23(Suppl 1)**:39–43.

25 Schulman CC, Sassine AM. Neoadjuvant hormonal deprivation before radical prostatectomy. *Eur Urol* 1993;**24**:450–455.

26 Gibbons RP, Jonsson E. Adjuvant radiation therapy following radical prostatectomy for pathologic stage C prostate cancer. *Eur Urol*. 1995;**27(Suppl)**:24–25.

27 Soloway MS, Sharifi R, Wood D, *et al*. Randomized comparison of radical prostatectomy alone or preceded by androgen deprivation for cT2B prostate cancer. J Urol 1995;**153(4)**:391A.

28 Zelefsky MJ, Leibel SA, Burman CM, *et al*. Neoadjuvant hormonal therapy improves the therapeutic ratio in patients with bulky prostatic cancer treated with three-dimensional conformal radiation therapy. *Int J Rad Oncol Biol Phys* 1994;**29(4)**:775–761.

29 Lee F, Bahn DK, McHugh TA, *et al*. US-guided percutaneous cryoablation of prostate cancer. *Radiology* 1994;**192**:769–776.

CHAPTER 11

TREATMENT OPTIONS FOR LOCALLY ADVANCED DISEASE

As previously emphasized, there has been a progressive downward migration in stage with which patients with prostate cancer present in many developed countries since the advent of PSA testing, which is especially marked in the USA. Worldwide, however, not inconsiderable numbers of men still present with, or subsequently develop, locally advanced malignant prostatic disease.

The term 'locally advanced prostate cancer' implies a tumour that is no longer gland-confined, but which has metastasized neither to local lymphatics nor to other more distant sites such as bone. It has to be conceded that the imprecisions of local staging methods, other than pathology after surgery, can result in either overstaging or, more commonly, understaging of this T3NoMo (Stage C) disease. In general, patients with locally advanced prostate cancer have biopsies revealing either moderately well-differentiated, or poorly differentiated, adenocarcinoma, a considerably elevated PSA (>20 ng/ml), a transrectal ultrasound suggesting extracapsular disease, together with negative pelvic CT and radionuclide bone scans.

Unfortunately, as in so many areas in the treatment of prostate cancer, there have been few properly conducted, randomized, long-term trials to help us advise patients and their families with any certainty of their best therapeutic option in this situation. Indeed, it is in the management of locally advanced disease where medical opinions are often most sharply divergent. In such circumstances *all* treatment options should be carefully and clearly discussed with the patient. It must also be remembered that many men with locally advanced prostate cancer are old (some very old) and, as for gland-confined disease in those with a limited life expectancy, observation only by "so-called" watchful waiting may be a legitimate option.

The currently available treatment options are discussed below.

SURGERY ALONE

Although the results of several series of surgical therapy by radical retropubic prostatectomy for T3NoMo cancers have revealed prolonged survivals[1,2], most patients with extracapsular prostatic cancer will eventually succumb to disseminated disease (unless, of course, they die of something else first). Because of this, the risks of morbidity or mortality following radical extirpative surgery are generally considered unjustified for these patients.

SURGERY AFTER HORMONAL DOWNSTAGING

In an attempt to improve cure rates in patients with T3NoMo prostate cancer, some urologists have employed a period of pre-operative androgen ablation therapy. This has usually taken the form of 3 months of an LHRH analogue, in combination with an antiandrogen such as flutamide, prior to radical retropubic prostatectomy. Several phase 2 studies of this approach have been reported, usually compared against historical 'controls'[3,4]. The conclusions that such 'hormonal downstaging' reduces the incidence of positive margins of course implies that the tumour in these patients has somehow shrunk back to be confined within the prostate. The improbability of such a phenomenon makes it mandatory that the long-term results of several currently recruiting randomized phase 3 studies are awaited before such manoeuvres become part of standard urological practice.

EXTERNAL-BEAM RADIOTHERAPY ALONE

Although, theoretically, it might appear that patients with locally advanced prostatic cancer without evidence of distant metastases might be ideal candidates for external-beam radiotherapy, in fact it is in these circumstances that the limitations of this modality of treatment are most apparent. Although reasonable survival data have been reported[5], there has been a worryingly high incidence of post-treatment prostatic biopsies showing viable adenocarcinoma cells[6]. Those patients whose biopsies do show residual cancer cells also appear to have a poorer prognosis than biopsy-negative individuals (due to the development of metastatic disease). Of more clinical importance, perhaps, is the failure of radiotherapy to reliably suppress PSA to within the normal range. A persistently raised or rising PSA after radiotherapy worries both the patient and clinician alike, and usually suggests the need for further adjunctive therapy. The frequent failures of external-beam radiation as monotherapy in such circumstances have provided the impetus for using neo-adjuvant endocrine therapy with radio-therapy.

EXTERNAL-BEAM RADIOTHERAPY PLUS HORMONAL THERAPY

The theory that lies behind the combination of hormonal ablation and external-beam radiation maintains that the pre-treatment reduction of tumour burden by endocrine ablation will increase the chances of 100% kill of cancer cells by irradiation. The prospect that the clones of hormonally insensitive cells that eventually result in hormonal relapse could be thus irradicated is certainly appealing. However, it could equally well be argued that the reduction in cell division rate that occurs after hormonal ablation might in fact render the cells *more* rather than *less* radio-resistant. The answer to these questions must await the results of several randomized studies that are currently in progress, and until then this treatment strategy should be regarded as investigational.

INTERMITTENT ANDROGEN SUPPRESSION THERAPY FOR LOCALLY ADVANCED PROSTATE CANCER

The ablation of testicular function for the palliative treatment of locally advanced prostate cancer was first attempted in the 1930s with orchidectomy[7]. This proved much less effective than surgical orchidectomy, which was introduced nearly a decade later by Huggins and Hodges[8]. No other treatment exists that equals or surpasses androgen ablation in checking the growth of prostate cancer and reducing its volume in 60–80% of patients. However, for reasons that remain uncertain, the cell-death process induced by androgen ablation

fails to eliminate the entire malignant-cell population. Another limitation of conventional androgen ablation is that it may conceivably increase the rate of progression of prostate cancer to an androgen-independent state[9]. In contrast, theoretically progression may be delayed by intermittent androgen suppression, a form of ablative therapy delivered in pulses[10]. For this reason, intermittent androgen suppression therapy is now being evaluated by Bruckovsky and others.

Three Essential Mechanisms of Regulation

Intermittent androgen suppression may work because essential mechanisms that determine the size of the prostate can be activated to check malignant growth[11]. As discussed in Chapter 4, normal control over cell divisions is established by three levels of androgen-mediated regulation: positive effects on initiation of DNA synthesis and cell proliferation, negative or inhibitory effects which limit the number of cells in the prostate, and apoptosis, an androgen-repressed process of programmed cell death which actively eliminates cells from the prostate when androgens are withdrawn.

Androgen Dependence and Independence

Androgen dependence is the clinical manifestation of apoptosis after androgen withdrawal in both normal and malignant tissues In fact, in the early stages of prostate cancer, only the negative type of regulation is missing[12]. Since the other two mechanisms are still functional, androgen ablation has the double effect of triggering apoptosis and inhibiting DNA synthesis and cell proliferation. Even in malignancy, the ability to undergo apoptosis is acquired as a feature of differentiation under the influence of androgens; thus in the absence of androgens, it is impossible for dividing cells to differentiate and become pre-apoptotic again[10,12]. This may explain why recurrent tumour growth is characterized by androgen independence.

In attempting to avert or delay progression to the androgen-independent state, it has been hypothesized that if malignant cells which survive androgen withdrawal are forced into a normal pathway of differentiation by androgen replacement, then apoptotic potential might be restored – hence setting the stage for a further response to therapeutic androgen withdrawal (**11.1**).

Experimental Observations

The androgen-dependent Shionogi carcinoma tumour model responds to androgen ablation in a manner strongly reminiscent of prostate cancer. When the parent tumour is transplanted into a male mouse, it grows with a short doubling time, regresses almost completely after castration, and recurs in an androgen-independent state[10]. Intermittent exposure of the parent Shionogi carcinoma to androgens has been carried out experimentally by transplanting the tumour into a succession of male mice, each of which was castrated when the estimated tumour weight was approximately 3 g. After the tumour regressed to 30% of the original weight, it was transplanted into the next non-castrated male. This cycle of transplantation and castration-induced apoptosis was successfully repeated four times before growth became androgen-independent during the fifth cycle[10]. The mean time to androgen independence of 147 days compared to 51 days after one-time castration was in keeping with a retarding effect of cyclical therapy on tumour progression.

Intermittent Androgen Suppression in Clinical Practice

With the advent of antiandrogens (such as Casodex and flutamide) and of LHRH agonists (including leuprolide acetate and goserelin acetate), new methods of androgen suppression which mimic the effects of orchidectomy by lowering the intranuclear concentration of dihydrotestosterone by 80% or more have become available. Emphasis has been placed on the combined use of such agents[13,14]; however, little attention has yet been given to their reversibility of action, the significance of which is potentially far-reaching. The possibility of a full recovery from therapy makes it possible to alternate a patient between periods of treatment and no-treatment. When the patient is off-treatment, the function of the testes and the concentration of serum testosterone slowly return to normal, over a period of 8–14 weeks. In response to this incremental androgenic stimulus, atrophic cells may be recruited into a normal pathway of differentiation where the risk of progression is small. With the associated movement through the division cycle, the cells become pre-apoptotic again, making it possible to repeat androgen deprivation therapy (**11.1**).

When to Interrupt Therapy?

A decrease of serum PSA to a stable nadir in a normal range, or a decreasing level, is an important aspect of the response to therapy[15,16]. If the serum PSA remains above 4 ng/ml between 24–32 weeks of treatment, it has been found that the median survival time is only 18 months[16]. On the other hand, if the serum PSA is below 4 ng/ml between 24–32 weeks of therapy, the median survival time is much greater at 40 months[17]. Only those patients whose serum PSA has reached a stable or decreasing value in a normal range at 24 and 32 weeks should be considered eligible for studies of intermittent androgen suppression with interruption of the therapy at around 36 weeks.

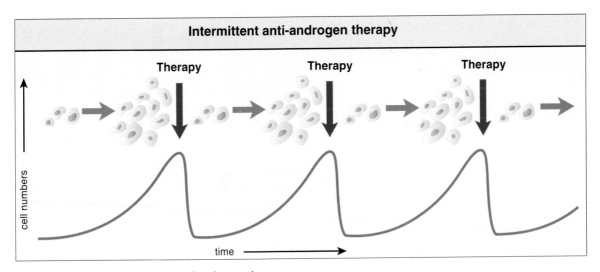

11.1 The concept of intermittent anti-androgen therapy.

When to Resume Therapy?

In patients with advanced prostate cancer, the serum PSA at the time of diagnosis may range in value from the upper limit of the normal range to a level of several thousand ng/ml. In those patients with a pre-treatment serum PSA below 20 ng/ml, the second cycle of treatment may be started when the serum PSA increases to the pre-treatment level again. If the serum PSA at presentation is greater than 20 ng/ml, the second cycle of therapy is started when the serum PSA increases to approximately 20 ng/ml. Following these guidelines, up to 5 cycles of therapy have been administered by Bruchovsky's group before there has been evidence of developing androgen-independence[18].

Applications of Intermittent Androgen Suppression

In theory, intermittent androgen suppression should be suitable for the long-term management of not only locally advanced prostate cancer, but also incompletely excised or locally recurrent prostate malignancy. Quality of life for the patient may potentially be improved with reduced toxicity from medication, recovery of sexual function and normal sense of well-being. There are also substantial potential cost savings.

Whether intermittent androgen suppression and its effects on tumour progression alter survival in an beneficial or adverse way is unknown; however, both time to progression and survival in a small number of patients with metastatic prostate cancer so far are similar to the expected results with continuous androgen ablation[17]. More information will become available from randomized trials of intermittent androgen suppression which are currently in the planning stages.

MANAGEMENT OF COMPLICATIONS FROM LOCALLY ADVANCED DISEASE

Patients with locally advanced prostate cancer are prone to either present with, or subsequently develop, local complications that severely affect the quality of life. The most common of these are bladder outflow obstruction with eventual acute or chronic urinary retention. Haematuria from tumour infiltration of the prostatic urethra or bladder base may also be troublesome. Although transurethral resection (TUR) of the obstructing and/or bleeding tissue is usually feasible, caution should be exercised in these circumstances because there is a higher incidence of urinary incontinence after TURP for malignant as opposed to

benign prostatic obstruction. This phenomenon is conventionally ascribed to infiltration of the distal urinary sphincter by malignant tissue, but, in fact, may be the result of technical difficulties caused by the loss of anatomical landmarks.

An alternative approach to the management of urinary retention due to prostate cancer is to employ androgen ablation therapy (usually with an LHRH analogue or bilateral orchidectomy) during an extended period of catheterization. On removal of the catheter after three months has elapsed, the majority of patients are able to void, although many probably remain obstructed[19]. A recent study randomized patients presenting with malignant prostatic obstruction to either TURP or hormonal therapy and catheterization, and found similar outcomes in both groups, but a lower incidence of incontinence in the conservatively managed cohort[20].

Many patients, however, are understandably reluctant to endure a three-month period of catheterization

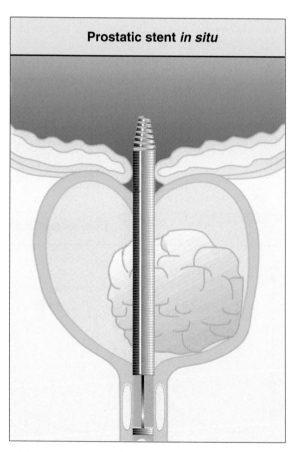

11.2 Porges Urospiral™ *in situ* relieving obstruction due to locally advanced prostatic tumour.

while the prostatic shrinkage is taking place. In such circumstances, it may now be legitimate to place a temporary intraurethral stent – such as a Porges 'Urospiral'™ (**11.2**, see also **11.3**) – to permit restoration of normal voiding over this time. However, problems with stent migration, urethral discomfort and lower urinary tract infection occur not uncommonly, and careful follow-up is mandatory.

Management of Malignant Obstruction of the Ureters due to Prostate Cancer

Locally advanced prostate cancer may also produce unilateral or bilateral ureteric obstruction (**11.4**). This may be due either to direct malignant infiltration of the ureters at the bladder base, or to compression by enlarged lymph nodes within the pelvis.

The former scenario may make management by retrograde insertion of double-pigtail ureteric stents (**11.5**) technically impossible, because of difficulties visualizing the ureteric orifices when infiltrated by

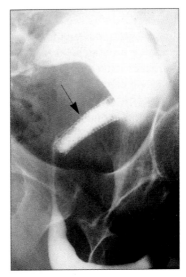

11.3 A cystogram showing a patient with a locally extensive prostate cancer voiding through a Urolume™ intra-prostatic stent (arrowed). (Courtesy of Dr David Rickards.)

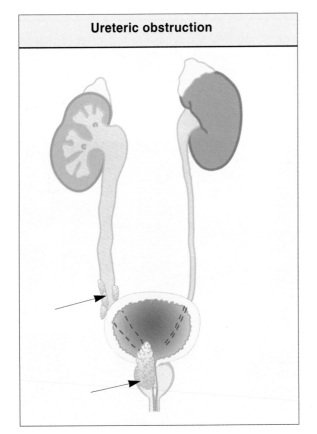

Ureteric obstruction

11.4 Ureteric obstruction in prostate cancer may occur at the level of the vesico–ureteric junction or at the pelvic brim due to lymph-node enlargement (arrowed).

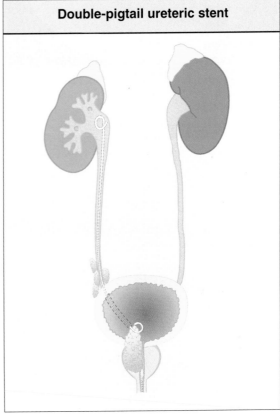

Double-pigtail ureteric stent

11.5 A double-pigtail ureteric stent may be inserted retrogradely.

malignant tissue. A way around this problem is to enlist the help of the radiologists in antegrade stent insertion (**11.6**); often a guide wire can be negotiated through the obstruction under radiographic control. Another option is to place a percutaneous nephrostomy or bilateral nephrostomies, to preserve renal function, while a response to either hormonal manip-

ulation and/or external-beam radiotherapy is awaited (**11.7**). Those elderly patients, however, who develop malignant bilateral ureteric obstruction after, or in spite of, hormonal manipulation, are usually best managed palliatively without percutaneous nephrostomies, since the quality of the short period of life prolongation achievable by these means is usually poor.

Other Problems Associated with Locally Advanced Prostatic Malignancy

In certain circumstances a bulky, locally advanced prostatic cancer may impinge posteriorly on the rectum (**11.8**). This development may result in the patient complaining of tenesmus and a sensation of incomplete rectal emptying. As the tumour continues to advance, severe constipation may develop, with eventual large-bowel obstruction. If all conservative measures fail, it is occasionally necessary to create a defunctioning colostomy in these unfortunate individuals.

CONCLUSIONS

Locally advanced prostate cancer often produces debilitating local symptoms that can markedly diminish the individual's quality of life. Correct management for the patient depends upon a combination of staging that is as accurate as possible, and an informed

11.6 Antegrade passage of a guide wire to allow placement of a double-pigtail stent. (Courtesy of Dr David Rickards.)

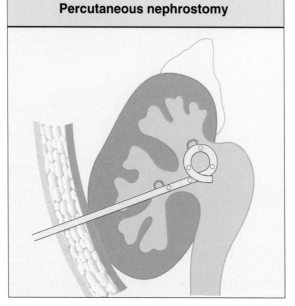

11.7 Percutaneous nephrostomy to relieve ureteric obstruction.

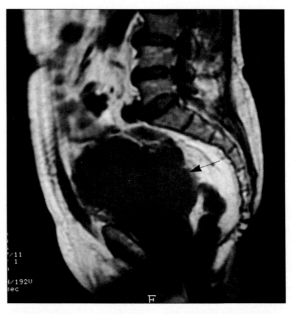

11.8 An MRI scan showing a locally extensive prostate cancer (arrowed) compressing the rectum posteriorly.

discussion with the individual and his family about the safety and efficacy of available treatment options. Until the results of randomized studies comparing various treatment options are available, the choice of therapy will continue to depend greatly on the personal experience of the urologist handling the case and the individual preferences of the patient and his immediate family.

REFERENCES

1 Catalona WJ, Bigg SW. Nerve-sparing radical prostatectomy: Evaluation of results after 250 patients. J Urol 1990;**143**:538–544.

2 deKernion JB, Neuwirth H, Stein A, et al. Prognosis of patients with stage D1 prostate carcinoma following radical prostatectomy with and without early endocrine therapy. J Urol 1990;**144**:700–703.

3 Flamm J, Fisher M, Holil W, et al. Complete androgen deprivation prior to radical prostatectomy in patients with stage T3 cancer of the prostate. Eur Urol 1991;**19**:192–195.

4 Labrie F, Dupont A, Gomez JL, et al. Beneficial effect of combination therapy administered prior to radical prostatectomy. J Urol 1993;**149(Abstract)**:348A.

5 Bagshaw MA. Radiation therapy for cancer of the prostate. In: Skinner DG, Lieskovsky G, (eds.) Diagnosis and Treatment of Genito-urinary Cancer. Philadelphia: W B Saunders, 1988; 425–445.

6 Freiha FS, Bagshaw MA. Carcinoma of the prostate: results of post-irradiation biopsy. Prostate 1984;**5**:19–23.

7 Sharifi R, Kiefer J. History of endocrine manipulation in the treatment of carcinoma of the prostate – who was first? J Endocrinol Invest 1987;**10(Suppl 2)**:91.

8 Huggins C, Hodges CV. Studies of prostatic cancer: I Effect of castration, oestrogen and androgen injections on serum phosphates in metastatic carcinoma of the prostate. Canc Res 1941;**1**:293–297.

9 Bruchovsky N, Lesser B, Van Doorn E, et al. Hormonal effects on cell proliferation in rat prostate. Vitamin Horm 1975;**33**:61–102.

10 Akakura K, Bruchovsky N, Goldenberg SL, et al. Effects of intermittent androgen suppression on androgen-dependent tumours: apoptosis and serum prostate specific antigen. Cancer 1993;**71**:2782–2790.

11 Bruchovsky N. Androgens and antiandrogens. In: Holland JF, Frei III E, Bast RC, et al. (eds.) Cancer Medicine. Philadelphia: Lea & Febiger, 1993;884–896.

12 Bruchovsky N, Brown EM, Coppin CM, et al. The endocrinology and treatment of prostate tumour progression. In: Coffey DS, Bruchovsky N, Gardner WA Jr, et al. (eds.) Current concepts and approaches to the study of prostate cancer. Progress in clinical and biological research. New York: Alan R. Liss Inc., 1987;348–387.

13 Crawford ED, Eisenberger MA, McLeod DG, et al. A controlled trial of leuprolide with and without flutamide in prostatic cancer. N Engl J Med 1989;**321**:419–424.

14 Denis L, Murphy GP. Overview of phase III trials on combined androgen treatment in patients with metastatic prostate cancer. Cancer 1993;**72(Suppl)**:3888–3895.

15 Miller JI, Ahmann FR, Drach GW, et al. The clinical usefulness of serum prostate specific antigen after hormonal therapy of metastatic prostate cancer. J Urol 1992;**147**:956–961.

16 Bruchovsky N, Goldenburg SL, Akakura K, et al. Luteinizing hormone-releasing hormone agonists in prostate cancer: Elimination of flare reaction by pretreatment with cyproterone acetate and low-dose diethylstilboestrol. Cancer 1993;**72**:1685–1691.

17 Goldenberg SL, Bruchovsky N, Gleave ME, et al. Intermittent androgen suppression in the treatment of prostate cancer. J Urol 1994;**151**:240A.

18 Goldenberg SL, Bruchovsky N, Gleave ME, et al. Intermittent androgen suppression in the treatment of prostate cancer: a preliminary report. Urology 1995;**45(5)**:839–845.

19 Hampson SJ, Davies JH, Charig CR, et al. LHRH analogues as primary treatment for urinary retention in patients with prostatic carcinoma. Br J Urol 1993;**71**:583–586.

20 Thomas DJ, Babaji VJ, Coptcoat MJ, et al. Acute urinary retention secondary to carcinoma of the prostate. Is initial channel TURP beneficial? Proc Roy Soc Med 1992;85:318–319.

CHAPTER 12

MANAGEMENT OF METASTATIC DISEASE

Unfortunately, despite the trend to earlier diagnosis already referred to, many patients with prostate cancer still present with either bony and/or soft tissue metastases. Others develop disseminated disease in spite of the best curative endeavours employed at a stage when the disease was still localized.

The mainstay of therapy for metastatic prostate cancer generally involves androgen deprivation, to which an initially favourable response will be seen in around 70–80% of patients. Almost inevitably, however, disease progression ('hormone escape') occurs eventually, due to the clonal selection of hormone-independent cancer cells. In this respect, there is now mounting evidence that, at least in some patients, the addition of an antiandrogen at an early stage to achieve so-called maximal androgen blockade (MAB) may significantly delay clinical disease progression and also prolong overall survival. When progression does eventually occur, and this is now usually heralded by a rise in serum PSA values, there is an understandable desire to implement effective second-line therapy. Unhappily, such manoeuvres do not always meet with success, although a number of new approaches are currently under evaluation. Contrary to popular belief, metastatic prostate cancer is often a lethal condition – 70% or so of patients dying *from*, rather than *with*, the disease within 5 years of diagnosis.

METHODS OF ANDROGEN DEPRIVATION

Bilateral Orchidectomy

The most cost-effective way of inducing permanent androgen deprivation is to undertake either bilateral orchidectomy or bilateral subcapsular orchidectomy (**12.1**). The procedure can be accomplished easily as a day case under a light general or regional anaesthetic, or even under local anaesthesia. The morbidity is low, and there are no concerns about either tumour flare or subsequent patient compliance. However,

many patients find the concept of surgical castration both worrisome and distasteful, and when offered the choice of either this or a luteinizing hormone-releasing hormone (LHRH) analogue, the majority (78% in one study) will now elect for the medical rather than surgical option[1]. The main side-effects of bilateral orchidectomy are minor local complications, such as haematoma formation and wound infection, as well as loss of libido and erectile impotence, and hot flushes. The psychological and cosmetic stigmata of castration can perhaps be reduced by performing the subcapsular excision of only the functional part of the organs, leaving a nubbin of residual testicular tissue on each side. A clinical response, usually manifested by a relief of bone pain, and rapid decline in serum PSA values, is seen in around 75% of patients treated by this means. The procedure is, of course, irreversible.

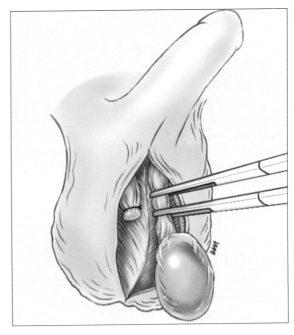

12.1 Bilateral orchidectomy is accomplished through a midline scrotal incision.

Administration of LHRH Analogues

Soon after the decapeptide structure of LHRH was elucidated, work began to develop LHRH analogues. These were synthesized by substitution or modification of one or more of the ten constituent amino acids. The result has been to produce superactive agonists which possess a prolonged duration of action. The administration of these agents causes an initial stimulation of LH and FSH production with a resultant rise in serum testosterone to 140–170% of basal levels. Within 2 weeks, however, LHRH analogues cause an inhibition of LH and FSH release, and a subsequent suppression of testosterone secretion similar to that seen after surgical castration (**12.2**). Chronic administration of LHRH analogues makes the pituitary resistant to further stimulation by endogenous LHRH, and the production of testicular androgens is therefore prevented. However, adrenal secretion of the 5% or so of residual androgens is under control of ACTH, and is therefore unaffected by the administration of LHRH analogues.

The most commonly used LHRH analogues are goserelin acetate, buserelin and leuprolide acetate. Goserelin acetate 3.6 mg and leuprolide acetate 3.75 mg are available as monthly copolymer and depot suspension formulations respectively. Goserelin is administered by subcutaneous injection, usually into the abdominal wall through a wide bore needle (**12.3**), leuprolide is given intramuscularly through a conventional needle. A new long-acting 10.8 mg depot formulation of goserelin has now been developed and is effective when administered on a three-monthly basis[2,3].

Discomfort at the injection site can be minimized by the prior administration of local anaesthetic. The principal side-effect is the potential 'tumour flare' that can accompany the initial rise in plasma testosterone. This may manifest itself as an increase in either bone pain or obstructive voiding symptoms; occasionally, catastrophic spinal-cord compression, due presumably to transient androgen stimulation of tumour cells, may develop. Because of this, some feel it is advisable that LHRH analogues be administered concomitantly with an antiandrogen for the first 4 weeks of therapy to prevent this devastating adverse effect. Other side-effects of LHRH analogues are those generally of androgen deprivation, namely, loss of libido, erectile impotence and reduction of body hair, similar to that seen after surgical castration.

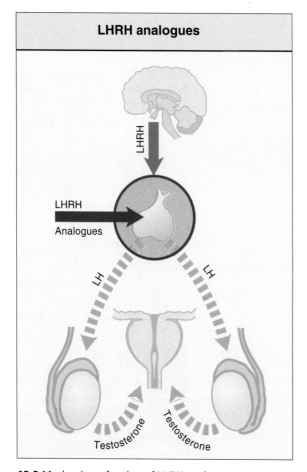

12.2 Mechanism of action of LHRH analogues.

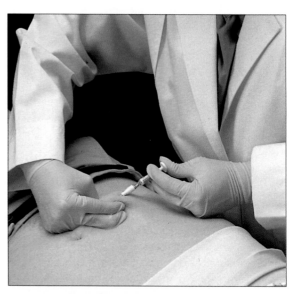

12.3 Depot preparations of LHRH analogues (such as goserelin acetate) are injected into the subcutaneous tissues of the abdomen; leuprolide acetate depot suspension is given intramuscularly.

Several large studies have demonstrated the equivalence of diethylstilboestrol (DES), leuprolide, goserelin and orchidectomy in terms of both time to progression and overall survival[4-6].

Monotherapy with LHRH Analogues versus Maximal Androgen Blockade (MAB)

Although numerous studies have confirmed that an initial response may be obtained in 70–80% of patients with metastatic prostate cancer, this remission following alteration of the hormonal milieu is unfortunately not usually maintained in the longer term. The average time to subsequent tumour progression is less than 18 months, with a mean overall survival time of around 18–28 months. Huggins and Scott[7] were the first to recognize the ephemeral nature of the response to testicular androgen ablation, and, as early as 1945, attempted to treat relapsing patients surgically by bilateral adrenalectomy. Unfortunately, adrenal replacement therapy was less than adequate in these early days and no patient survived longer than 4 months. None the less, with their classic studies, these Nobel-prize winning researchers not only laid the framework for most future clinical studies of prostatic cancer, but also first raised the important question of the role of adrenal androgens in sustaining tumour growth once testicular androgens have been withdrawn.

While most urologists have been content to manage their patients with advanced prostatic cancer by testicular androgen ablation (using either bilateral orchidectomy or depot preparations of LHRH analogues such as leuprolide or goserelin acetate), for more than a decade Labrie and co-workers have been urging the therapeutic addition of an antiandrogen to suppress a postulated stimulatory effect by residual androgens of adrenal origin. This manoeuvre, they have argued, enhances initial response rates, delays the development of subsequent androgen independence, and improves both time to progression and overall survival. However, this approach of 'total androgen blockade' has important implications in terms of additional drug toxicity and in adding considerably to the health economic burden of the disease. Therefore, the evidence for and against this contention – both in the laboratory and more importantly from clinical trials – needs to be carefully weighed before clinicians in general are encouraged to adopt this approach.

Evidence from Animal Models for a Contribution by Adrenal Androgens

The mechanisms by which prostatic cancer cells develop the ability to grow despite androgen depletion are still incompletely understood, but may involve a series of events including mutations of androgen receptors, the over-expression of oncogenes (which encode various mitogenic growth factors), and the deletion of tumour-suppressor genes. Critical from the viewpoint of the efficacy, or otherwise, of total androgen blockade are the androgen requirements of the developing tumour.

In the Shionogi mammary-tumour cell line, which is very sensitive to DHT, Labrie and Veilleux[8] have, by plating single cells, identified clones of cells that are extremely sensitive to the growth stimulating effects of low concentrations of androgens. Stimulation of cell division of different clones of Shionogi cells by DHT were seen in vitro at very low concentrations, ranging from 10^{-8} to 10^{-11} molar. The same group of workers have also demonstrated stimulatory effects of adrenal androgen precursors on ventral prostate weight, as well as androgen-dependent gene expression in the castrated rat model. Importantly, these effects were observed at plasma concentrations of DHEA and androstenedione comparable to those found in the sera of adult castrated men[9].

By contrast, other workers using alternative androgen-sensitive cell lines have not been able to identify clones exhibiting sensitivity to such low levels of androgens or androgen precursors. They have also argued that the development of androgen insensitivity in vitro and in vivo is more likely to be the result of the natural selection of cell lines which can flourish independently of any need for androgen stimulation. In such circumstances, more complete suppression of androgen levels by total androgen blockade might be anticipated to be of little or no beneficial use.

Ellis and Issacs[10] performed a series of experiments and compared the effects of partial versus complete androgen ablation in the treatment of rats with the Dunning 3327H (well-differentiated) and 3327R (poorly differentiated) tumour. Using control groups, tumour-bearing rats were treated with either orchidectomy alone or with orchidectomy and cyproterone acetate, a progestational antiandrogen. There was no significant difference in either tumour growth or overall survival between the two groups, but cyproterone is not the most effective antiandrogen.

CLINICAL STUDIES OF MAXIMAL ANDROGEN BLOCKADE

For a number of reasons, prostatic cancer is an inherently difficult tumour to study. As previously discussed, histological foci of prostate cancer have been demonstrated to be present in up to 30% of men over the age of 50, yet clinical cancer only develops in 7–9% of individuals; unequal inclusion of cases of low-volume, well-differentiated carcinomas in single-arm studies or in trials of competing therapies may therefore lead to misleading information concerning their efficacy. The doubling time of prostate cancer is often slow (6 months to 4 years, or even more) compared with other tumours, which means a long observation period is necessary before the results of clinical studies can be correctly evaluated. Finally, the behaviour of individual prostatic tumours – even when extensive metastases are present – is rather unpredictable; some respond for prolonged periods to androgen withdrawal while others progress relentlessly in spite of all therapy. Large numbers of patients of similar disease status must therefore enter each arm of any study, as unequal stratification of patients will certainly result in significant bias. Many of the reports relating to efficacy of total androgen withdrawal can be criticized for the inadequate numbers of patients studied, the unequal stratification of comparison groups and, especially, the lack of maturity of data in terms of period of patient observation at the time of reporting. All these factors may account for the apparent disparity of results, not only in this but in many other areas of prostate cancer research.

As discussed before, the main protagonists of total androgen blockade have been Labrie and co-workers from Quebec, Canada, who have produced a series of publications on the subject[11-13]. Unfortunately, much of their data were based on phase II observational studies which have employed rather weak criteria by which objective response to therapy is defined. Protocols have not always been strictly followed; for example, in one prospective multicentre study of 94 patients with histologically proven prostatic adenocarcinoma[14] treated by castration or by LHRH agonist plus an antiandrogen, the castration arm was discontinued when 4 of 7 patients entering this arm of the study died after 11, 16, 17 and 29 months respectively. The remaining group of 87 patients who received combined treatment were reported to have an initial response of 100% and a probability of a continuing positive response at 2 years of 81%. Of the 8 (11.9%) patients in this arm

who relapsed, only 1 perished from prostate cancer and 3 from other causes. These results compare extremely favourably with standard therapy in which only testicular androgens are ablated – where progression may be anticipated in roughly one third of patients within one year – and were initially greeted with considerable scepticism by the urological community. However, further impetus towards a more rigorous evaluation of the clinical effect of maximal androgen blockade came from the demonstration that as much as 10–15% of intraprostatic DHT remains after medical or surgical castration[15]. Moreover, Harper et al. confirmed that, in fact, adrenal androgens may be responsible for as much as 15–20% of total intraprostatic DHT[16].

In response to the claims of Labrie and co-workers, a prospective, randomized placebo-controlled trial was established with the assistance of the National Cancer Institute (NCI) in 1984 in the USA. The protocol was simple in its design, comparing leuprolide 1 mg subcutaneously per day with placebo, against leuprolide 1 mg subcutaneously per day plus flutamide 250 mg tds in patients with metastatic cancer of the prostate confirmed on radioisotope bone scan. Crossover from placebo to flutamide was allowed at the first signs of tumour progression. Six hundred and three patients from 93 contributing institutions were recruited within 18 months[17] and results stratified according to the severity of the disease and patient performance status at the time of presentation. Overall median, progression-free survival favoured the group receiving flutamide (16.5 months versus 13.9 months), as did overall survival (35.6 months for the flutamide arm versus 28.3 months for the placebo arm) (**12.4**).

In the subset analysis, patients with good performance status and minimal disease on bone scan (defined as absence of disease in ribs, long bones, skull, or soft tissues other than lymph nodes), who were treated with total androgen blockade at diagnosis (41 patients in each arm), experienced a longer time to objective progression (48 months for the flutamide arm, 19 months for the placebo arm) and prolonged overall survival (median 61 months versus 42 months) (**12.5**). The majority of patients fell into the category of good performance status, but with severe disease (241 patients in each arm). In this group, median time to progression was prolonged by 3 months through the addition of flutamide (16 months versus 13 months) and overall survival was enhanced by 6 months in the combination therapy group. Diarrhoea was the main side-effect reported, more frequently by the flutamide group (13.6% of subjects)[18,19].

Not all studies of various alternative regimes of maximal androgen blockade compared with monotherapy have confirmed such unequivocal advantage. Denis[20], however, has reported an update of EORTC data showing improved cancer-specific survival in a EORTC study comparing goserelin acetate implants (Zoladex) plus flutamide against orchidectomy, amounting to some 7 months' advantage for the combination therapy (**12.6**). Keuppens *et al.*[21] had previously reported a benefit in the flutamide group in delaying the time to first progression (p=0.004) but, at that stage, survival advantage had not been seen, perhaps because of the lack of maturity of the study.

In a Canadian study in which a different non-steroidal antiandrogen, nilutamide (Anandron), was compared with an identical placebo plus bilateral orchidectomy[22], it was found that although there was a delay in progression, no clear demonstration of improved survival was apparent. A similar double-blind placebo-controlled study involving 457 patients with metastatic disease has been reported by Janknegt[23]. Statistically significant differences were found in favour of orchidectomy plus nilutamide in complete or partial response (p < 0.001), and in cancer-related survival (p = 0.046), compared with patients treated by orchidectomy alone.

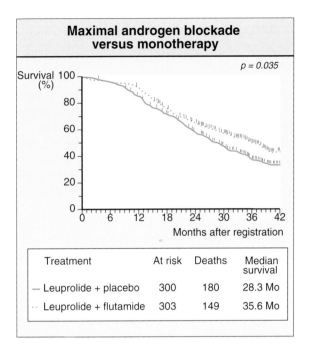

12.4 Kaplan–Meier survival curves of patients with metastatic prostate cancer treated with leuprolide alone versus leuprolide + flutamide 250mg tds (i.e. maximal androgen blockade)[17].

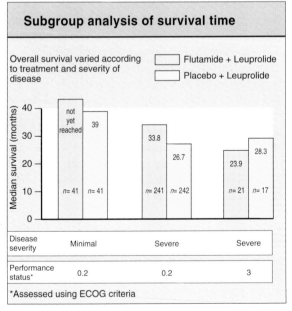

12.5 Differences in survival in patients with metastatic prostate cancer treated with LHRH analogue alone versus maximum androgen blockade[17].

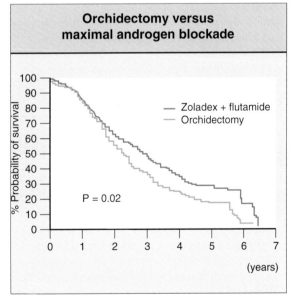

12.6 Duration of survival following either orchidectomy or maximal androgen blockade[20].

By contrast, several other studies have failed to demonstrate any definite benefit of maximal androgen blockade over monotherapy with either LHRH analogues or orchidectomy. A large prospective, randomized trial comparing goserelin acetate (3.6 mg sc/month) and flutamide to orchidectomy alone did not confirm any significant difference in subjective response rate, time to disease progression or overall survival in 571 evaluable subjects after a mean follow-up of two years[24]. Another study combining the EORTC data mentioned above[21] with a similar Danish study allowing an evaluation of altogether 591 patients treated by either goserelin acetate plus flutamide or orchidectomy also failed to demonstrate any significant difference in overall survival, although time to progression and the specific death rate from prostate cancer were delayed by the introduction of combination therapy[25].

At the time of reporting of the latter study, however, the median follow-up had again only just reached 2 years. It must be remembered that such a short follow-up period may mask the potential benefit of maximal androgen blockade since the patients dying early in the study period are likely to be those with severe disease (i.e. heavy tumour burden) and poor performance status, in whom combination therapy is unlikely to confer very much benefit. As these combined data mature, therefore, as seems to be the case with the EORTC study[16], the curves in at least a subset of patients with less advanced disease may separate.

Since the advent of serum PSA determination in patients with prostate cancer, a powerful additional tool has been acquired by which the efficacy of various treatment options can be compared. To date, only a few studies have reported the comparative extent of PSA decline with maximal androgen blockade compared with that seen with orchidectomy or LHRH analogues. However, Smith and colleagues[26] reported recently that 98% of 411 prospectively treated patients with metastatic prostate cancer had a decrease in PSA levels with a median reduction of 97.7% 3 months after randomization to leuprolide plus nilutamide or leuprolide plus placebo. A greater proportion (76%) of those on maximal androgen blockade had normalization of their PSA value within three months than those treated with leuprolide alone (52%). The difference was statistically significant ($p < 0.0001$).

One possible explanation for the delay in tumour progression and survival advantage seen in at least some reports of maximal androgen blockade is that LHRH analogues, when employed without a con-comitant antiandrogen, produce a transient surge of LH release and a consequent rise in testosterone levels. This may result in a 'tumour flare'[27], which usually manifests itself as acute exacerbation of bone pain, though occasionally devastating spinal cord compression may occur. This may be prevented by commencing with LHRH analogues and antiandrogens simultaneously. However, such a tumour flare does not occur when the method of ablation of testicular androgens is bilateral orchidectomy. As mentioned above, the addition of an antiandrogen to bilateral orchidectomy also seems to improve results in some studies[22,23]. A more recent NCI sponsored study of orchidectomy plus flutamide versus orchidectomy alone is currently recruiting, and should throw further light on this question.

OTHER METHODS OF ACHIEVING MAXIMAL ANDROGEN BLOCKADE

Although the majority of data reviewed above suggest that the combination of either leuprolide or goserelin acetate (or alternatively bilateral orchidectomy) with either flutamide or nilutamide, and more recently the once/day antiandrogen Casodex, may provide some additional benefit to monotherapy (which ablates only testicular androgens) in at least a subgroup of patients, there are several other pharmacological agents available that seem potentially capable of achieving similar effects, although data on these are less complete. Several alternative therapeutic options are discussed below:

Diethylstilboestrol (DES), which has the advantage of being very cheap, has unfortunate and well-documented cardiovascular toxicity at either 5 mg/day or 3 mg/day dosage. At 1 mg/day, however, this does not appear to be too great a problem, although at this dosage serum testosterone levels are not reliably suppressed into the castrate range[28]. However, the EORTC Protocol 30805, in which patients were randomized to either 1 mg DES/day or bilateral orchidectomy +/– cyproterone acetate, showed no differences in either survival or cardiovascular thromboembolic events[29]. These data suggest that randomized studies of an antiandrogen plus low-dose diethylstilboestrol (DES) versus the more expensive option of an LHRH analogue plus an antiandrogen may be worthwhile, although the side-effects of DES induced gynaecomastia are still liable to be troublesome, even at 1 mg/day (**12.7**). Gynaecomastia may be prevented by single-dose radiotherapy to the pectoral area. Others have advocated the addition of one aspirin/day to reduce cardiovascular effects of DES, but there are currently no data to confirm the efficacy of such a manoeuvre.

Cyproterone acetate and *megestrol acetate* are steroidal antiandrogens (**12.8**), both of which have marked progestational activity which inhibits LH release from the pituitary and produces castrate levels of testosterone; they also compete with testosterone and dihydrotestosterone (DHT) for androgen receptor sites. However, if used as monotherapy, there tends to be a gradual increase in testosterone values with chronic usage (as a result of escape of pituitary inhibition), and

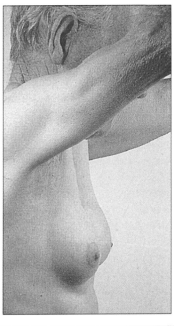

12.7 Gynaecomastia induced by treatment of prostate cancer with diethylstilboestrol.

they are probably not as effective as DES or orchidectomy. There are few data available yet of their value in combination with LHRH analogues or orchidectomy. Side-effects of cyproterone include an increased risk of thrombosis with cardiovascular consequences as well as an increased tendency towards diabetes. Disturbances of liver function have been reported, including four recent cases of hepatocellular carcinoma among long-term cyproterone users[30,31].

Flutamide, a non-steroidal antiandrogen (**12.9**), has been used by some urologists as monotherapy for metastatic prostate cancer. However, it has not yet been approved by any regulatory authority for this indication, and most experts have contended that flutamide should usually be used only in conjunction with medical or surgical castration. Calculations based on known affinities of DHT and flutamide for the androgen receptor suggest that when flutamide is used as monotherapy, it leaves at least 40% of androgen receptor sites available for binding by DHT; when combined with castration, however, only 5% of DHT is available to the androgen receptor. Unlike most other agents that are active against prostate cancer, flutamide when used alone does not appear always, or even usually, to affect libido and potency adversely. Diarrhoea, however, is not uncommon, and gynaecomastia and breast tenderness also occur, presumably because of an increased aromatization of testosterone to oestradiol. These latter effects are not seen when flutamide is combined with an LHRH analogue. In a recent study, Boccon-Gibot[32] compared flutamide 250 mg administered 3 times/day to bilateral orchidectomy

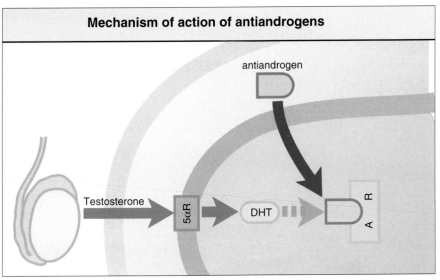

Mechanism of action of antiandrogens

antiandrogen

Testosterone → 5αR → DHT ▌▌▌ → A R

12.8 Mechanism of action of antiandrogens which interfere with DHT interaction with androgen receptors.

in 104 patients with newly diagnosed metastatic prostate cancer. In those patients whose PSA was less than 120 ng/ml at inclusion the two arms produced similar responses, not only in terms of PSA suppression, but also for progression-free survival.

Nilutamide (Anandron) is a non-steroidal, pure antiandrogen which is similar in structure to flutamide. In contrast to cyproterone acetate, it is devoid of progestational and antigonadotrophic properties. It competes with testosterone and DHT at the androgen receptor, not only at the level of the prostate, but also at the hypothalamo–pituitary complex (where androgens exert their negative feedback effect); as a result, LH secretion is enhanced and, in the presence of intact testes, testosterone biosynthesis is increased. However, because of the presence of the antiandrogen, the effects of the rising testosterone at the receptor level are blunted. Its main value seems to be in combination with an LHRH analogue, as has already been discussed[22,23]. Side-effects of nilutamide include gastrointestinal symptoms, anaemia, disturbances of light/dark adaptation and alcohol intolerance.

Casodex (bicalutamide) is a new, non-steroidal antiandrogen that binds to the androgen receptor on the rat prostate with about 2% of the affinity of DHT, but roughly four times the affinity of hydroxyflutamide (12.10). Unlike flutamide, Casodex does not cause a marked elevation in serum LH and testosterone in rats

or dogs, and has a much longer half-life[33]. A steady state is reached after about a month of therapy. Phase II clinical trials revealed reasonable efficacy of Casodex when used as monotherapy in patients with metastatic prostate cancer, as judged by both acid phosphatase and PSA level decline. The most frequent side-effects were breast tenderness, gynaecomastia and hot flushes, but the incidence of hot flushes was lower in those receiving Casodex monotherapy (9%) than those treated by orchidectomy (41%) or combination with LHRH analogue (49%). In man, in contrast to the preclinical studies in other animals, Casodex, like flutamide, appears to elevate serum testosterone levels somewhat, due to central antagonism of T receptors in the hypothalamo–pituitary complex – there is a consequent increase of LH secretion[34]. However, Casodex's long half-life of about one week enables maintenance of high serum concentrations and allows once daily dosing; moreover, serum testosterone concentrations in patients treated with Casodex rarely exceed the normal range that the drug must antagonize.

Phase III studies of Casodex at both 50 mg and 150 mg per day dosages have been undertaken in North America and Europe[35]. Casodex 50 mg monotherapy dose revealed statistically significant inferior efficacy results in comparison with castration (12.11). Large Phase III randomized trials comparing Casodex 150 mg

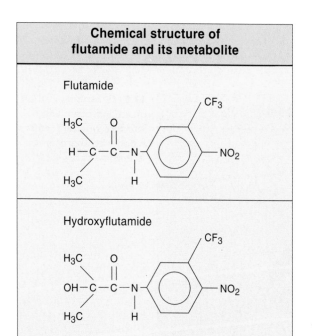

Chemical structure of flutamide and its metabolite

Flutamide

Hydroxyflutamide

12.9 Structure of flutamide and its major metabolite.

Chemical structure of Casodex

12.10 Structure of the antiandrogen Casodex (bicalutamide).

monotherapy with either the LHRH analogue, Zoladex, or orchidectomy are in progress. Casodex's profile of low toxicity and once/day oral dosage regime makes it a strong candidate for the future – especially since there is evidence of benefit for Casodex monotherapy in sexual interest and function at some timepoints in some studies.

In the context of combination therapy, a multicentre, randomized, double-blind study of Casodex 50 mg + LHRH analogue and flutamide 750 mg + LHRH analogue has recently been completed in North America. A total of 813 patients were recruited for a minimum follow-up of 6 months. Casodex–LHRH analogue therapy was associated with a significant improvement in time to treatment failure than the flutamide–LHRH analogue combination (p=0.005) (**12.12**). In all, 88 patients withdrew from treatment because of an adverse event: 32 from the Casodex–LHRH analogue arm and 56 in the flutamide–LHRH analogue arm. Diarrhoea was more frequently reported in patients treated with flutamide–LHRH analogue than Casodex–LHRH analogue (24% vs 10%, p<0.001) and was the most frequent adverse event leading to withdrawal (25 for flutamide–LHRH analogue and 2 for Casodex–LHRH analogue. Abnormal liver-enzyme test results were reported in both groups (25 for Casodex–LHRH analogue, 41 for flutamide–LHRH analogue) and the number of patients who had study therapy withdrawn was similar in both treatment groups (6 for Casodex–

LHRH analogue and 8 for flutamide–LHRH analogue)[36]. Assessment of quality of life questionnaires did not reveal any significant difference between the two treatment groups, but patients in both arms experienced a reduction in pain, improved physical capacity, better emotional well-being and more vitality. Casodex and Zoladex are trademarks, the property of Zeneca Limited.

Aminoglutethimide blocks the conversion of cholesterol into pregnenolone, thus inhibiting the production not only of testicular and adrenal androgens, but also of aldosterone, cortisol and oestrogens; it also inhibits peripheral aromatase activity. This blocking effect is accomplished by binding to the cytochrome P450 moiety of enzyme complexes. Replacement glucocorticoids must therefore be given with aminoglutethimide to avoid cortisol insufficiency, and to prevent the reflex rise of ACTH which would otherwise act to overcome the effects of chemical blockade. There are no currently available data on the use of aminoglutethimide as first-line therapy in metastatic prostate cancer, either used singly or in combination with an LHRH analogue. What data there are have mainly been accrued from patients with relapsed prostate cancer after primary treatment with ablation of testicular androgens. After the initial studies of Robinson *et al.* in 1974[37], a few other reports, mainly with subjective response rates, followed. At most, one third of patients obtained some benefit for only lim-

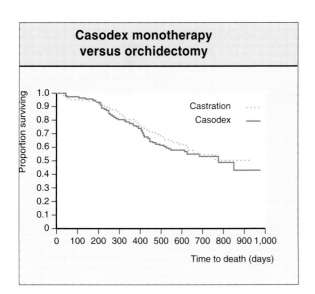

12.11 Phase III studies of Casodex 50 mg versus orchidectomy.

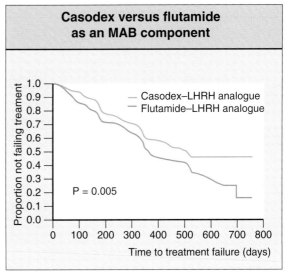

12.12 Kaplan–Meier probability of treatment failure in two alternative forms of maximal androgen blockade (MAB)[32].

ited periods of time from medical adrenalectomy by aminoglutethimide–cortisol combination therapy. Side-effects were troublesome and included lethargy, rash and drowsiness in a substantial number of patients. Two Australian studies reported around 20% subjective response rates in patients with prostate cancer in relapse, in 126 and 34 patients respectively, for reasonably prolonged periods[38,39]; however, the exact role of the additional cortisone supplements in achieving these results is unknown, since it has been shown that corticosteroids alone can produce some improvement in patients with advanced prostate cancer[40].

Ketoconazole, a synthetic imidazole dioxalane, is active against a number of fungi by virtue of its inhibitory effect on cytochrome P450. At higher doses than are necessary for fungicidal action, the same effect inhibits the C17-20 lyase biosynthesis in the adrenals, thereby reducing the production of adrenal androgens. In general, plasma glucocorticoids and mineralocorticoids are not affected, although there have been reports of adrenal insufficiency in debilitated patients treated with this medication. In patients with relapsed prostatic cancer treated with ketoconazole, around 50% subjective improvement but little objective improvement has been reported[41]. Side-effects at this high dosage, however, are common with this drug, particularly gastrointestinal toxicity, and,

more rarely but alarmingly, severe hepatoxicity; for this reason it is now rarely used.

Finasteride is a 4-aza steroid competitor of 5-alpha reductase – the enzyme that converts testosterone to DHT within the prostate (12.13). Several studies have confirmed that finasteride reduces serum DHT by 75% while maintaining testosterone levels, and results in significant regression of the benignly enlarged gland[42,43]. Geller et al.[44] have shown that finasteride results in a marked decline of intraprostatic DHT, but a rise in intraprostatic testosterone levels. Animal studies suggested that finasteride would have activity in prostatic cancer[45], and a pilot study in 28 patients with metastatic prostate cancer showed some declines in PSA, but less than seen after orchidectomy or treatment with an LHRH analogue[46]. However, in a randomized study of patients who had positive margins after radical prostatectomy, finasteride delayed the rise in PSA by around 18 months[47] (12.14). Finasteride is a competitive inhibitor of 5-alpha reductase; in contrast, other inhibitors, such as the new agent SK&F 105657, are thought to be uncompetitive inhibitors. A recent report of the use of this agent in androgen-responsive cell lines and in R-3327 tumour-bearing rats suggested some potentially useful anti-tumour activity[48]. However, at the time of writing, there have been no published phase II reports of the effect of this compound in patients. The appeal of a 5-alpha

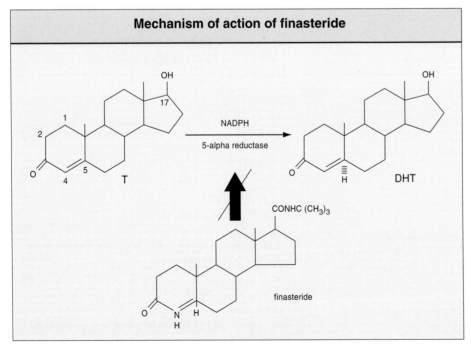

Mechanism of action of finasteride

NADPH

5-alpha reductase

T

DHT

CONHC(CH₃)₃

finasteride

12.13 Finasteride, a 5-alpha reductase inhibitor, competitively inhibits the conversion of testosterone to dihydrotestosterone (DHT).

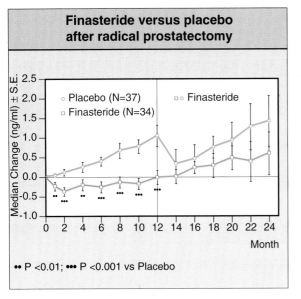

12.14 Effect of finasteride on serum PSA of patients who are found to be margin positive on histology after radical prostatectomy[47].

reductase inhibitor in this context is the very favourable toxicity profile compared with the agents discussed above; virtually the only side-effect seen with finasteride is a 3–5% incidence of impotence and loss of libido, which is reversible on discontinuing the drug. The hypothesis that a combination of a 5-alpha reductase inhibitor with an antiandrogen may be of some value is currently being evaluated in a randomized phase II study.

TIMING OF ENDOCRINE ABLATION THERAPY FOR METASTATIC PROSTATE CANCER

Traditionally, urologists have tended to favour deferred administration of hormonal manipulation in patients with advanced prostate cancer, often waiting until symptoms appear before acting medically or surgically to ablate testicular androgens. The rationale for this decision to defer therapy was to some extent based on the findings from Study I of the Veterans Administration Cooperative Urological Research Group (VACURG). In this study, when patients were randomized between immediate hormonal therapy and placebo therapy, with later hormonal therapy when they became symptomatic, there was no difference in average survival rates between the two groups[49]. Sarosdy[50] however, has re-

analysed the VACURG Study I data in detail, withdrawing the deaths due to cardiovascular events in the oestrogen-treated group and calculating cancer-specific death rates. These recalculations show that those who were treated initially with oestrogen therapy in fact fared better than those treated with placebo (3% cancer deaths in the oestrogen group versus 8.4% in the placebo group; p=0.008).

The studies of total androgen blockade mentioned above have now produced further evidence of the potentially deleterious effects of allowing metastases of prostatic cancer to progress unfettered until a considerable tumour burden eventually produces symptoms. The enhanced results (both in terms of time to progression and overall survival in a subgroup of patients with good performance status and minimal metastatic disease) in at least some studies[17,20,23] now provide further support for those advocating more prompt intervention in patients who present with M1 disease. The MRC Prostate Study Group has completed recruitment of over 800 patients with metastatic prostate cancer and has randomized them into immediate androgen ablation versus deferred therapy groups. As yet, however, the data are not mature enough to confirm a disease-specific survival advantage for one group over another, but the results of this study are anticipated by 1996.

CONCLUSIONS

The current gold standard – first-line therapy for metastatic prostate cancer – is androgen ablation by either bilateral orchidectomy or the use of LHRH analogues. However, Labrie's original hypothesis that androgen precursors secreted by the adrenal glands may play a role in maintaining prostate cancer growth and the escape of tumour cells from hormone control after ablation of testicular androgens is now gaining increasing scientific credence. The burden of evidence from a number of randomized, multicentre studies is that a subgroup of patients with good performance status and a reasonably restricted volume of metastatic disease may in fact remain in remission longer and have a more prolonged survival if treated by maximal androgen blockade rather than conventionally with LHRH analogues or orchidectomy alone. More work is needed to confirm these results, and much of the data needs more time to mature before final evaluation, as the economic implications for already overstretched healthcare budgets are not inconsiderable. However, the current position is that if we wish to offer the very best therapy to our patients, then maximal androgen blockade with an antiandrogen plus either an LHRH analogue or bilateral orchidectomy is now the recommended treatment in the fitter younger individuals who do not present with an unduly heavy burden of prostate cancer, and in whom eventual death from prostate cancer, rather than a comorbid condition, seems likely[51].

For the future, it should be possible to pre-identify (for example, by biochemical or morphometric means) the subgroup of patients in whom total androgen blockade, rather than orchidectomy or LHRH analogues alone, may produce a definite survival advantage. Moreover, there seems to be the promise of equally effective monotherapy by orally administered antiandrogens, which may obviate the need for either injections or surgery and also preserve potency and thereby quality of life. The challenge of confirming these suggestions may be added to the many others that face us as we strive to reduce the morbidity and mortality of this most prevalent disease of men beyond middle age.

REFERENCES

1 Cassileth BR. Patients' choice of treatment in stage D prostate cancer. Urology 1989;**33(Suppl 5)**:57–59.

2 Dijkman GA, Debruyne FMJ, Fernandez de Moral P, et al. A Phase III randomized trial comparing the efficacy and safety of the 3-monthly 10.8 mg depot of Zoladex with 3.6 mg depot in patients with advanced prostate cancer. Eur Urol 1994;**26(1)**:1–2.

3 Debruyne FMJ. Zoladex 10.8 mg depot for prostate cancer. J Urol 1995;**153**:448A.

4 Peeling WB. Phase III studies to compare goserelin (Zoladex) with orchidectomy and diethylstilbestrol in treatment of prostatic carcinoma. Urology 1989;**33**:45–52.

5 Leuprolide Study Group. Leuprolide versus diethylstilbestrol for metastatic prostate cancer. N Eng J Med 1984;**311**:1281–1286.

6 Debruyne FMJ. Long-term therapy with a depot luteinizing hormone-releasing hormone analogue (Zoladex) in patients with advanced prostatic carcinoma. J Urology 1988;**140**:775–777.

7 Huggins C, Scott WW. Bilateral adrenalectomy in prostate cancer. Ann Surg 1945;1031–1041.

8 Labrie F, Veilleux R. A wide range of sensitivities to androgens develops in cloned Shionogi mouse mammary tumour cells. Prostate 1986;**8**:293–300.

9 Labrie C, Simand J, Begin D. Conversion of precursor adrenal steroids into potent androgens in peripheral tissues. In: Labrie F, Lee F, Dupont A, (eds.) Early stage prostate cancer: diagnosis and choice of therapy. Amsterdam: Elsevier Science Publishers BV, 1989;1–21.

10 Ellis WJ, Issacs JT. Effectiveness of complete versus partial androgen withdrawal therapy for the treatment of prostate cancer as studies in the Dunning R-3327 system of rat prostatic adenocarcinomas. Canc Res 1985;**45**:6041–6045.

11 Labrie F, Dupont A, Belanger A. New approach in the treatment of prostate cancer: complete instead of partial withdrawal of androgens. Prostate 19;**4**:579–594.

12 Labrie F, Dupont A, Belanger A. Combination therapy with flutamide and castration (LHRH agonist or orchidectomy) in advanced prostate cancer: a marked improvement in response and survival. J Steroid Biochem 19;**23**:833–841.

13 Labrie F. Benefits of combination therapy with flutamide in patients relapsing after castration. Br J Urol 1988;**61**:341.

14 Labrie F, Dupont A, Belanger A, et al. Combination therapy with flutamide and castration (LHRH agonist or orchiectomy) in advanced prostate cancer: a marked improvement in response and survival. J Steroid Biochem 1985;**23**:833–841.

15 Geller J, De La Vega DJ, Albert JD. Tissue dihydrotestosterone levels and clinical response to hormone therapy in patients with prostate cancer. J Clin Endocrinol Metab 1984;**58**:36–40.

16 Harper ME, Pike A, Peeling WB, et al. Steroids of adrenal origin metabolized by human prostate tissue both in vivo and in vitro. J Endocrinol 1984;**60**:117.

17 Crawford ED, Eisenberger MA, McLeod DG, et al. A controlled trial of leuprolide with and without flutamide in prostatic cancer. N Engl J Med 1989;**321**:419–424.

18 Crawford ED, Nabors WL. Total androgen blockade: American experience. Urol Clin North Am 1991;**18**:55–63.

19 Mayer FJ, Crawford ED. Optimal therapy for metastatic prostate cancer. In: Hendry WF, Kirby RS, (eds.) Recent advances in urology/andrology. Churchill Livingstone, 1993;159–176.

20 Denis LD, Carneiro de Moura JL, et al. Goserelin acetate and flutamide versus bilateral orchiectomy: a phase III EORTC trial (30853). Urology 1993;**42(2)**:119–129.

21 Keuppens F, Denis L, Smith P. Zoladex and flutamide versus bilateral orchidectomy. A randomized phase III EORTC 30853 study. Cancer 1990;**66**:1045–1057.

22 Canadian Anandron Study Group. Total androgen blockade in the treatment of metastatic prostate cancer. Seminar Urol 1990;**8**:159–162.

23 Janknegt RA. International Anandron Study Group: Efficacy and tolerance of a total androgen blockade with Anandron and orchidectomy. A double-blind, placebo controlled multicentre study. J Urol 1991;**145**:425A.

24 Lunglmayr A. The international prostate cancer study group. A multicentre trial comparing the LHRH analogue Zoladex, with Zoladex plus flutamide in the treatment of advanced prostate cancer. Eur Urol 1990;**18(suppl3)**:28–29.

25 Iversen P, Sucini S, Sylvester R. Zoladex and flutamide versus orchidectomy in the treatment of advanced prostate cancer. A combined analysis of two European studies EORTC and DAPROCA 86. *Cancer* 1990;**66**:1067–1073.

26 Smith JA, Crawford ED, Lange PH. PSA correlation with response and survival in advanced carcinoma of the prostate. *J Urol* 1991;**145**:384A.

27 Kahan A, Delriu M, Amor B. Disease flare induced by D-Trp-6-LHRH analogue in patients with metastatic prostate cancer. *The Lancet* 1984;971–972.

28 Shearer RJ, Hendry WF, Sommerville IF. Plasma testosterone, an accurate monitor of hormone treatment in prostate cancer. *Br J Urol* 1973;**45**:668–671.

29 Robinson MRB. Complete androgen blockade: the EORTC experience comparing orchidectomy versus orchidectomy plus cyproterone acetate versus low dose stilboestrol in the treatment of metastatic carcinoma of the prostate: Proceedings of the Second International Symposium on Prostate Cancer. *Prostate Cancer Part A, Research, Endocrine Treatment and Histopathology* New York, Alan Liss, Inc 1987;383–390.(Abstract)

30 Watanabe S, Yamasaki S, Tanae A, *et al.* Three cases of hepatocellular carcinoma among cyproterone users. *Lancet* 1994;**344**:1567–1568.

31 Ohri SK, Caer JAR, Keane PF. Hepatocellular carcinoma and treatment with cyproterone acetate. *Br J Urol* 1991;**67**:213–221.

32 Boccon-Gibot L, Fournier G, Bottet P, *et al.* Flutamide versus orchidectomy in patients with metastatic prostate cancer. XI *Congress of the* EAU 1994;**Abstracts Book**:13.

33 Furr BJA, Valcaccia B, Curry B. ICI 176334. A novel non-steroidal peripherally selective antiandrogen. *J Endocrinol* 1987;**113**:R7–R9.

34 Kennealey GT, Furr BJA. Use of the non-steroidal antiandrogen Casodex in advanced prostatic cancer. *Urol Clin North America* 1991;**18**:99–110.

35 Kaisary V. Current clinical studies with a new steroidal antiandrogen, Casodex. *Prostate* 1994;**5S**:27–33.

36 Shelhammer P, Sharifi R, Block N, *et al.* A controlled trial of bicalcutamide (Casodex) versus flutamide each in combination with LHRH analogue therapy in patients with D_2 prostatic carcinoma. (In press.)

37 Robinson MRG, Shearer RJ, Fergusson JD. Adrenal suppression in the treatment of carcinoma of the prostate. *Br J Urol* 1974;**46**:555–559.

38 Murray R, Pitt P. Aminoglutethimide in the treatment of advanced prostate cancer. In: Murphy G, Khoury S, Kuss R, *et al.* (eds.) *Prostate Cancer.* New York: A.R. Liss, 1987;275–282.

39 Harnett DR, Raghavan D, Caterson I. Aminoglutethimide in advanced prostate carcinoma. *Br J Urol* 1987;**59**:323–327.

40 Plowman PN, Perry LA, Chard T. Androgen suppression by hydrocortisone without aminoglutethimide in orchidectomized men with prostate cancer. *Br J Urol* 1987;**59**:255–257.

41 Pont A. Long-term experience with high dose ketoconazole therapy in patients with D2 prostate carcinoma. *J Urol* 1987;**137**:902–904.

42 Gormley GJ, Stoner E, Bruskewitz RC, *et al.* The effect of finasteride in men with benign prostatic hyperplasia. *N Engl J Med* 1992;**327**:1185–1191.

43 Kirby RS, Vale J, Bryan J, *et al.* Long-term urodynamic effects of finasteride in benign prostatic hyperplasia: a pilot study. *Eur Urol* 1993;**24**:20–26.

44 Geller J. Effect of finasteride, a 5-alpha reductase inhibitor on prostate tissue androgens and prostate specific antigen. *J Clin Endocrinol Metab* 1990;**71**:1552–1555.

45 Brooks JR, Berman C, Nguyen H, *et al.* Effect of castration, DES, Flutamide, and the 5-alpha reductase inhibitor MK906, on the growth of the Dunning rat prostatic carcinoma, R-3327. *Prostate* 1991;**18**:215–217.

46 Presti JC, Fair WR, Andriole G, *et al.* Multicentre, randomised, double-blind, placebo-controlled study to investigate the effect of finasteride (MK-906) on stage D prostatic cancer. *J Urol* 1992;**148**:1201–1204.

47 Andriole GL. Finasteride induced PSA reductions in patients with early stage prostate cancer. *J Urol Abstract* 1994;**151**:450A.

48 Lamb JC, Levy MA, Johnson RK, *et al.* Response of rat and human prostatic tumours to the novel 5-alpha reductase inhibitor, SK&F 105657. *Prostate* 1992;**21**:15–34.

49 Veterans Administration Cooperative Urological Research Group. Carcinoma of the prostate: treatment comparisons. *J Urol* 1967;**98**:516–519.

50 Sarosy MF. Do we have a national treatment plan for stage D1 carcinoma of the prostate. *World J Urol* 1990;**8**:27–31.

51 Kirby RS. Is total androgen blockade now mandatory? *Rev Endocrine-Related Cancer* 1994;**42**:31–43.

CHAPTER 13

MANAGEMENT OF HORMONE-ESCAPED PROSTATE CANCER

Unhappily, as already described, unless some comorbid condition intervenes, virtually every advanced prostate cancer treated by androgen ablation will eventually 'escape' from the growth-restraining effects of low circulating androgen levels, and will show signs of disease progression. The mechanism for this hormone escape is almost certainly the clonal selection of androgen-independent cell lines (**13.1**). Now that serial PSA determination is readily available and commonly utilized for follow-up, 'PSA relapse' is frequently seen as an inevitable harbinger of clinical disease progression. This leaves the urologist and his or her patient in the position of knowing the worst and therefore wishing to employ second-line therapy before symptoms inexorably develop. Although the prognosis in these circumstances is generally still poor, there are now some manoeuvres that it may be helpful to institute.

VARIATIONS ON THE THEME OF ANDROGEN ABLATION

For those patients who have been managed initially by monotherapy (by either orchidectomy or LHRH analogues), the addition of an antiandrogen to neutralize the 5% or so of circulating adrenal androgens would seem logical. However, by the time hormone escape has occurred, this often has disappointingly little, if any, beneficial effect. Recently, the observation has been made that certain patients who have been managed from the outset with maximal androgen blockade may benefit from cessation of the antiandrogen[1]. In such circumstances, the rising serum PSA may be temporarily halted or reversed by flutamide withdrawal. Although this phenomenon is presently unexplained, it could be the result of an agonist effect of the antiandrogen on mutated androgen receptors in tumour cells.

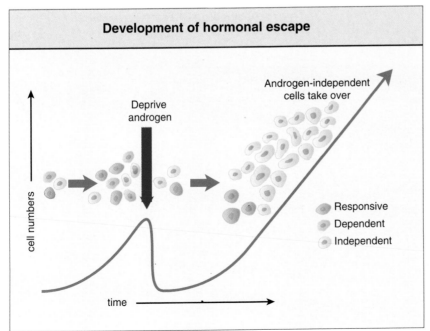

Development of hormonal escape

Deprive androgen

Androgen-independent cells take over

Responsive
Dependent
Independent

cell numbers

time

13.1 Clonal selection of androgen-independent cells resulting in hormonal escape.

This would be akin to the mild oestrogenic effect of the antioestrogen tamoxifen, which is sometimes seen in breast cancer, and which is probably due to structural mutation of oestrogen receptors in breast cancer cells. Flutamide withdrawal is such a simple and cost-effective measure that it should now be considered in situations of prostate cancer relapse in spite of maximum androgen blockade. Moreover, it must be borne in mind that if some new form of therapy is initiated at the same time as flutamide withdrawal, then any clinical or biochemical improvement seen may conceivably be incorrectly ascribed to the new drug rather than to the withdrawal of the original therapy.

Diethylstilboestrol

Another treatment strategy for relapsed prostate cancer is to introduce an oestrogen such as diethylstilboestrol (DES) at this stage. Although the major action of oestrogens in prostate cancer is at the hypothal-amo–pituitary level, there is also evidence of a direct cytotoxic effect on prostate cancer cells, conceivably by direct inhibition of DNA polymerase. Evidence for the efficacy of DES in this context, however, is virtually all anecdotal, since randomized studies have seldom proven practical in the situation of disease relapse.

A recent study in experimental animals has suggested that hormonal escape itself might be delayed by the introduction of oestrogens[2]. The side-effects of oestrogens, including gynaecomastia, deep vein thrombosis (4%), and other cardiovascular complications, usually preclude the use of DES as first-line therapy. In situations of hormonal relapse, however, where life expectancy is so limited, a therapeutic trial may be indicated, and it has been suggested, but not yet proven, that the cardiovascular side-effects can be minimized by additional dosing with 50 mg of aspirin per day.

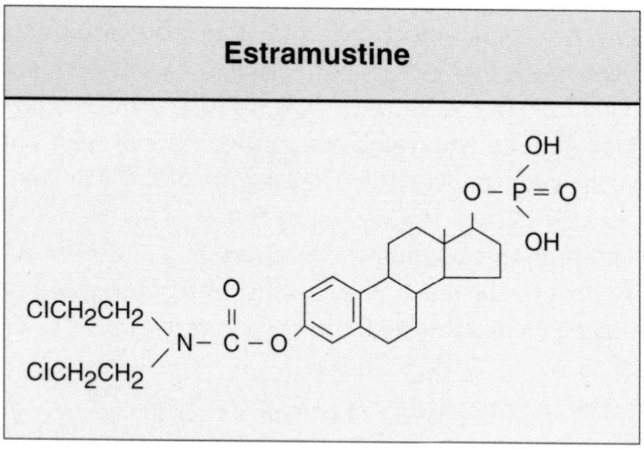

Estramustine Phosphate

Another drug with oestrogenic effects that is currently making something of a comeback is estramustine phosphate (EMP). This agent is a combination of nitrogen mustard linked to a phosphorylated estradiol (13.2). EMP is rapidly dephosphorylated in the body to its main metabolites, estramustine and estromustine[3]. Only 10% or so of these metabolites are hydrolyzed to estradiol and estrone, which act secondarily to depress testosterone levels (13.3). These oestrogenic steroid metabolites are present in considerably lower concentrations than those achieved with the standard doses of oestrogen used in the treatment of metastatic prostate cancer, and are not the

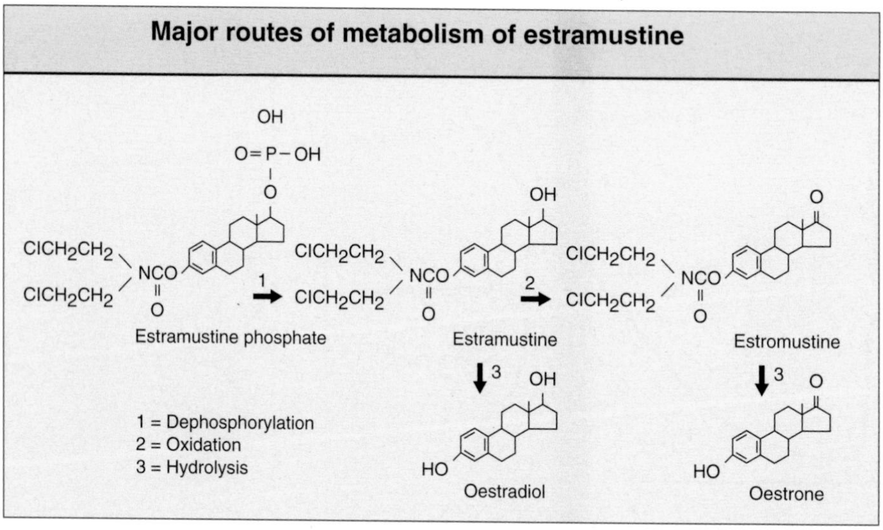

Estramustine

13.2 Chemical structure of estramustine.

Major routes of metabolism of estramustine

13.3 Metabolism of estramustine.

Estramustine phosphate → 1 → Estramustine → 2 → Estromustine

1 = Dephosphorylation
2 = Oxidation
3 = Hydrolysis

Oestradiol   Oestrone

primary mode of anti-cancer action of the drug. EMP cytotoxicity is mainly due to its ability to bind to microtubule-associated proteins (MAPs).

As discussed in Chapter 4, MAPs are essential to microtubule stability and microtubules are intimately involved in the cell cycle. Estramustine causes microtubules to disassemble, as well as preventing their *de novo* formation (**13.4**), thereby resulting in mitotic arrest during metaphase and cell death[4].

Estramustine appears to accumulate preferentially in the prostate; in one study, prostate biopsies showed concentrations of estramustine six times higher than those achieved in the plasma. In the relatively hormone-resistant human prostate cancer cell line DU 145, estramustine has been shown to inhibit cell growth[5,6]. Moreover, in a number of phase 2 and phase 3 trials of estramustine as second-line therapy, the drug has been shown to produce an overall subjective response rate of around 60%, and an objective response rate in 30–35% of patients (**Tables 13.1** and **13.2**). Toxicity can be a problem though, especially in the typically frail and elderly patient with hormone-relapsed cancer. Nausea, anaemia and granulocytopenia can all occur, any of which may necessitate the cessation of therapy.

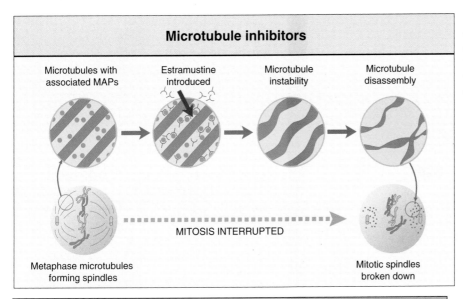

Microtubule inhibitors

Microtubules with associated MAPs — Estramustine introduced — Microtubule instability — Microtubule disassembly

MITOSIS INTERRUPTED

Metaphase microtubules forming spindles

Mitotic spindles broken down

13.4 The action of estramustine in dissassembling microtubules and thereby preventing cell division.

Table 13.1 Summary of selected phase II studies of estramustine in hormone-refractory prostate cancer

Reference	No. of patients	Objective response (%)
Benson *et al.* (1986)[32]	51	69
Chisholm *et al.* (1977)[33]	30	27
Fosså & Miller (1976)[34]	17	35
Jönsson *et al.* (1977)[35]	91	31
Küss *et al.* (1980)[36]	15	20
Leistenschneider & Nagel (1980)[37]	23	35
Lindberg (1972)[38]	22	27
Mittelman *et al.* (1976)[39]	44	18
Veronesi *et al.* (1982)[25]	27	74

Table 13.2 Phase III clinical trials of estramustine in hormone-refractory prostate cancer patients

Reference	Protocol	Treatment (no. of patients)	Objective response (%)
Murphy et al. (1977)[40]	NPCP Protocol 200	Estracyt (46) Streptozotocin (38) Standard therapy (21)	30 31 19
Soloway et al. (1981)[41]	NPCP Protocol 800	Estracyt (27) Estracyt + vincristine (19) Vincristine (34)	26 24 15
Soloway et al. (1983)[42]	NPCP Protocol 1200	Estracyt (40) Estracyt + cisplatinum (42) Cisplatinum (42)	18 33 21

Abbreviation: NPCP = National Prostatic Cancer Project

USE OF CYTOTOXIC AGENTS

Cytotoxic agents have often been tried in metastatic prostate cancer, either alone or in combination, both as primary therapy and in situations of hormonal relapse. Unfortunately, although partial responses may be obtained in some cases, in neither circumstance has the objective response rate been of sufficient magnitude to counter balance the toxicity often seen, which is often especially severe in this group of elderly men who have frequently received prior radiotherapy, and who also often have pre-existing bone marrow suppression due to bone metastases. The original problem of the lack of bidimensionally measurable disease in assessing the response to therapy has to some extent been overcome by the advent of quantitative PSA determination. However, as yet, not many reports of chemotherapeutic agents have included PSA data. The issue is further clouded by the fact that, not uncommonly, patients exhibit a 'mixed response'; for example, improvement in soft-tissue disease sites, but advancement in other areas, most commonly in bone metastases.

For several years, the National Prostatic Cancer Project (NPCP) has utilized criteria for response that were developed by their group which includes a category for 'stable disease' (SD) as evidence of a response to therapy[7]. By their definition, SD represents no evidence of disease progression during the initial 12 weeks of therapy. Survival analysis of patients with SD appeared to be comparable to those who had evidence of partial response (PR); both groups survived significantly longer than those who did not respond. For these reasons, patients with SD are often considered in the category of 'responders', together with those exhibiting evidence of partial response. Since the tumour-doubling time of many prostatic cancers is notoriously slow, even in advanced disease, it may well be that the apparent disease stabilization observed over 12 weeks was not in fact due to the treatment itself. Inclusion of patients with SD in responder groups may therefore falsely inflate apparent treatment response rates.

Experience with Single Agents and Multidrug Combinations in Single Arm Studies

The experience with single-agent chemotherapeutic regimes in prostate cancer has not been especially encouraging. The methodological problems already alluded to make it difficult to estimate the exact level of antitumour activity of most drugs. The marked variability of reported response rates probably reflects different methodologies as well as widely varying patient selection criteria.

Because of the disappointing response rates to single-agent chemotherapy, a number of investigators have employed multidrug regimens in patients with metastatic prostate cancer. Unfortunately, the number of complete or even partial responses has generally remained low; moreover, the toxicity associated with multidrug therapy is usually greater than that of single-agent treatment.

Prospective Randomized Studies of Chemotherapy in Endocrine-Resistant Prostate Cancer

For obvious reasons, randomized studies of chemotherapy are easier to interpret than single-arm studies. They also usually serve to evaluate more clinically relevant end-points, such as time to treatment failure and overall survival. Some of the more important randomized studies are summarized in **Table 13.3**. In virtually all of them, the differences between the chemotherapy arm and standard therapy, which usually consisted of various palliative measures including

treatment with corticosteroids, analgesics, and palliative radiation to painful metastases, were negligible. In several large NPCP studies of multidrug regimes, the Kaplan–Meier survival curves constructed for both arms were virtually identical (**13.5**).

THE USE OF GROWTH FACTOR INHIBITORS

The accumulating evidence suggesting that growth factors, including epidermal growth factor (EGF), insulin-like growth factor (IGF), platelet-derived growth factor (PDGF), as well as fibroblast growth factor (FGF), may be involved in the development and progression of prostate cancer has stimulated researchers to evaluate the effect of the growth factor inhibitors, such as suramin, in patients with metastatic prostate cancer (**13.6**). Suramin is a polysulphonated napthylurea analogue of tryptan blue, with several important biological activities including growth factor inhibition[8].

Treatment	No. evaluable/ entered	Complete and partial response	Stable disease	Median survival (weeks)
Table 13.3 National Prostatic Cancer Project: randomized trials in prostate cancer				
NPCP study 100[42,43]				
Cyclophosphamide	41	4	4	47
5-Fluorouracil	33	4	4	44
Standard therapy	36	0	0	38
NPCP study 200[44,45]				
Estramustine	46/54	3	3	26
Streptozotocin	38/46	0	0	25
Standard therapy	21/25	0	0	24
NPCP study 300[46]				
Cyclophosphamide	35/39	0	9	27
DTIC	55/68	2	13	40
Procarbazine	39/58	0	5	31
NPCP study 700[47]				
Cyclophosphamide	43/47	3	12	41
MeCCNU	27/38	1	7	22
Hydroxyurea	28/40	2	2	19
NPCP study 800[48]				
Estramustine	27/38	1	6	26
Vincristine	29/42	1	4	22
Estramustine + Vincristine	34/41	0	7	32
NPCP study 1200[49]				
Estramustine	40/50	0	7	38
Cisplatinum	42/51	0	9	28
Estramustine + Cisplatin	42/48	0	14	40

Chemotherapy versus standard therapy

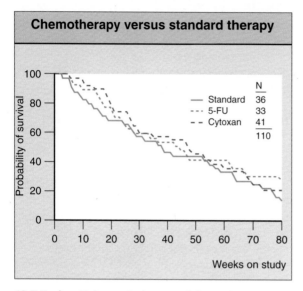

13.5 Kaplan–Meier survival curves of chemotherapy versus palliative measures only in patients with hormone-escaped metastatic prostate cancer. 5-FU = 5-fluorouracil. (Reproduced from Oesterling et al.[50])

Growth factor inhibitors

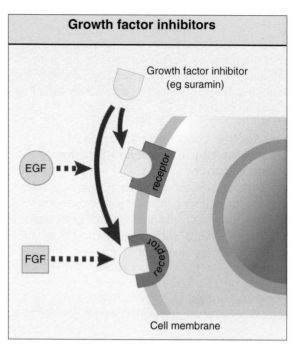

13.6 Mechanism of action of growth factor inhibitors such as suramin.

As discussed in Chapter 4, growth factors are involved in the pathogenesis of many cancers because malignant cells become the endogenous producers of polypeptide growth stimulators. Therapeutic interruption of this so-called autocrine loop has been most extensively investigated in systems dependent on PDGF. Human PDGF is a 30 000 molecular weight protein that is a mitogen to connective tissue-derived cells. The B chain of PDGD is virtually identical to part of the transforming protein v-sis of simian sarcoma virus (SSV), which suggests that a PDGF-like factor mediates cell transformation. When added to SSV-transformed human fibroblasts, suramin causes a reversible and dose-dependent reversion to the normal phenotype. Suramin can also interfere with the binding of insulin-like growth factor (IGF) to its receptors[9,10]. Unlike members of the EGF and FGF families, which are for the most part produced and act locally in tissues, IGF-I and IGF-II are produced both locally and systemically. IGF-I is released from the liver under the stimulation of growth hormone, and is the key mediator of growth-hormone effects. Prostatic cancer cells in tissue culture respond to insulin and its related peptides, and the blocking effect of suramin on IGF receptors may therefore account for some of its activity in metastatic prostate cancer.

Clinical trials to evaluate the effects of suramin in hormone-refractory prostate cancer began in 1988[11]. The drug was administered to patients as a continuous infusion to a target plasma level of 300 µg/ml. Of the 38 patients that entered this trial, 17 had measurable soft-tissue disease and the rest bone metastases alone. Thirty-three percent of the patients with soft-tissue metastases demonstrated shrinkage of deposits but more than 50% of those with bone secondaries did so. Seventy per cent had significant relief of bone pain and more than half had a greater than 50% decline in their serum PSA. The magnitude of the pre-treatment PSA was an important predictor of outcome: of those patients whose pre-treatment PSA was <100 ng/ml 70% had a greater than 75% decline in PSA in response to suramin. By contrast, only a quarter of patients with pre-treatment PSA values >100 showed similar responses. From this, it was concluded that the effectiveness of suramin was limited dramatically by the extent of the tumour burden.

Other preliminary reports from the USA of the use of suramin in prostate cancer have also been encouraging[12]. However, although some remissions have been documented, in general the side-effect profile of this agent is insufficiently clean for it to gain general acceptance for the treatment of this condition; skin rashes, prolonged bleeding time, keratopathy and neuromuscular toxicity have all been encountered. Many patients report paresthesiae involving the lower extremities and a syndrome of fever and chills, and more severe neurotoxicity with progressive peripheral neuropathy may also occur. Adrenal insufficiency and increased susceptibility to infections are also significant clinical problems with this agent. Growth factor inhibitors that are more specific to the prostate are eagerly awaited for deployment in patients with relapsing prostate cancer.

Taxol

The diterpine Taxol (paclitaxel, Mead Johnson, Princeton NJ), which is a natural product of the plant *Taxus brevifolia*, seems to hold the promise of some useful activity in hormone-refractory prostate cancer[13] (**13.7**). This compound has a unique mechanism of action, with high-affinity binding to polymerized microtubules at a site distinct from those identified for colchicine, vinblastine or estramustine (**13.4**). Recently, Taxol has been demonstrated to possess an ability to inhibit the invasiveness of an *in vitro* human prostate cancer cell line, and to inhibit the growth and metastatic potential of human prostate cancer xenografts[14].

A phase II study looking at paclitaxel in advanced, hormone-refractory carcinoma of the prostate was conducted by Roth *et al.*[15] Twenty-three patients (with bidimensionally measurable disease) were treated with paclitaxel 135–170 mg/m^2 by 24-hour IV infusion, every 21 days for a maximum of 6 cycles. In 21 evaluable patients, there was 1 partial response (4.3%) lasting 9 months. Four other patients with radiographically stable disease had minor reductions in the serum PSA of 16–24%. Eleven patients (47.8%) had stable disease, and progressive disease developed in 9 patients (39.1%) during therapy. The median survival was 9 months.

Leukopenia was generally the dose-limiting toxicity, with 13% of patients having Grade 3 and 61% having Grade 4 toxicity. Granulocytopenic fever developed in 26% of patients. The study concluded that in the setting of hormone-refractory prostate cancer and bidimensionally measurable disease, paclitaxel at this dosage has limited clinical activity.

Hudes *et al.*[16] conducted a phase 1 pharmacological study of a 96-hour infusion of paclitaxel combined with estramustine (600 mg/m^2 D$_1$–D$_2$) every 3 weeks in 18 patients with refractory tumours. Patients had received a median of 2 prior chemotherapy regimens. Paclitaxel was administered at a dose of 80–140 mg/m^2.

Objective responses occurred in 2 out of 2 patients with measurable hormone-refractory prostate cancer, and the authors concluded that such activity merits further investigation.

Retinoids and Prostate Cancer

Another interesting group of compounds with regard to the treatment of hormone-refractory prostate cancer are the retinoid derivatives of vitamin A. Within the nucleus retinoids act as transcription regulators, generally inhibiting growth and promoting epithelial-cell differentiation. Fenretinide (N-4-Hydroxyphenylretinamide) has been shown to be cytotoxic to both rat and human prostate cancer cells *in vitro*. Using various angiogenesis inhibition assays, it was demonstrated that fenretinide not only inhibited angiogenesis but also endothelial cell motility and tubule formation[17]. The potential for retinoids as chemopreventive agents in prostate cancer is discussed in Chapter 14.

Liarozole

Liarozole acts mainly by inhibiting the breakdown of retinoic acid, thus increasing retinoic acid levels. Retinoic acid is one of the principal endogenous com-

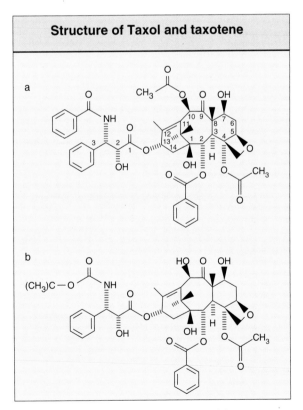

Structure of Taxol and taxotene

a

b

13.7 Molecular structure of (**a**) Taxol and (**b**) taxotene.

pounds that control growth and differentiation of epithelial cells. Besides their anti-proliferative and differentiation-inducing potencies, retinoids have important antitumoural activities. These have been demonstrated in acute promyelocytic leukaemia, as well as in solid tumours such as lung cancers and squamous cell carcinomas of both the head and neck and the skin.

Normally, retinoic acid is metabolized by means of a cytochrome P450-mediated hydroxylase enzyme system; this system is inhibited by liarozole (**13.8**). A further biological activity of liarozole is as an aromatase inhibitor, preventing the peripheral conversion of testosterone to oestrogen. The biosynthesis of testosterone is also cytochrome P450-dependent. Liarozole causes a dose-dependent lowering of testosterone, and a rise in the precursors 17 alpha-hydroxyprogesterone and progesterone for at least 24 hours after a single dose of 300 mg. Unlike ketoconazole, however, liarozole does not significantly effect adrenal androgen levels.

In experimental animals, liarozole has shown antitumoral effects in both androgen-dependent and androgen-independent prostate cancers[18]. The compound is now being evaluated in patients suffering clinical relapse after previous androgen-depletion therapy for prostate cancer. Early data suggests tolerance is acceptable overall, with most adverse events being mild to moderate, and mostly retinoid related (i.e. akin to hypervitaminosis A), such as dry mouth, itchy peeling skin, nausea, asthenia and fatigue. As more experience is gained, liarozole may have a place as therapy in metastatic disease, and perhaps even in locally advanced prostate cancer.

ROLE OF NEWER COMBINATION THERAPIES

As in the 1970s with testicular cancer, we are currently awaiting a major breakthrough in the therapy for hormone-relapsed metastatic prostate cancer. Now that some agents such as Taxol, suramin and liarozole are beginning to emerge with signs of useful activity, the possibility of improving efficacy with various combination therapies exists – e.g. growth factor inhibitors plus cytotoxic agents or retinoids; there seems to be plenty of scope for advancement in this area.

For example, the combination of estramustine with vinblastine has a logic, because both agents have distinctive and potentially synergistic effects as microtubule inhibitors. In vitro studies in the DU 145 human prostate cancer cell line demonstrated additive antimitotic effects. In recent clinical trials involving 82 patients, a PSA decline of more than 50% was achieved in 35 (43%) individuals. Moreover, 6 of 19 (32%) patients with bidimensionally measurable disease achieved a partial response. Vinblastine was usually given as a weekly, intravenous bolus of 4 mg/m^2 in combination with oral estramustine 10–15 mg/kg/day on days 1–42. Thereafter, treatment was repeated after a 2-week break if toxicity was acceptable and there was no disease progression. Toxicity was predominantly attributable to the estramustine, which causes cardiovascular side-effects such as venous and arterial thrombosis in up to 10% of cases; mild nausea and haematological disturbances were also reported in up to 50% of patients. Using a 50% PSA decrease as a clinical endpoint, Seidman et al.[19] also showed a promising response rate to this combination of between 30 and 50%.

Another interesting combination therapy is that of etoposide and estramustine. Etoposide is a topoisomerase II inhibitor that inhibits DNA replication directly at the level of the nuclear matrix. The results of etoposide used alone in prostate cancer have been disappointing.[20] However, in vitro etoposide combined with estramustine has been shown to inhibit growth in the human metastatic PC-3 cell line as well as the MAT-LyLu (MLL) rat prostate cancer cell line[21]. In a

---

Simplified pathway of retinoic acid catabolism

Retinoic acid

↓   4-hydroxylase (P450-dependent)

4-hydroxy-retinoic acid

↓

4-keto-retinoic acid

↓

↓   (at least partly P450-dependent)

↓

Polar metabolites

13.8 Retinoic metabolism is inhibited by liarozole.

phase 2 clinical trial, 20 patients with hormone-refractory prostate cancer were treated with estramustine 15 mg/kg/day and etoposide 50 mg/m^2/day, both taken orally for 21 out of 28 day cycles. Fifteen patients were available at the time of the first report, 9 of whom had measurable disease. A partial response was seen in 6 patients; the remaining 3 achieved stable disease. Toxicity consisted of nausea, granulocytopaenia and anaemia. All patients noted alopecia[22].

Other Forms of Palliation

In some circumstances, a short course of corticosteroids may be worth considering. It has been noted that this intervention may improve anaemia and weight loss and psychological well-being, but there are little scientific data to corroborate this contention.

Bone Pain

One of the most intractable and distressing problems encountered in hormone-escaped prostate cancer is bone pain associated with skeletal metastases. The usual analgesic agents are often of little efficacy in this situation. doses high enough to provide some relief are associated with unacceptable side-effects of sedation and confusion. The mechanisms for the often especially severe pain are incompletely understood. There may be an increase in intramedullary pressure and local invasion of endosteal, periosteal and marrow nerve endings. Obviously, pathologic fractures through tumour-affected bone should be excluded by local radiographs.

There is now some evidence that some patients with painful bony metastases may benefit from treatment with diphosphonates. Diphosphonates are pyrophosphate analogues that suppress bone resorption and mineralization by a direct influence on the activity of osteoclasts, and have been used in the treatment of Paget's disease, multiple myeloma and metastatic breast cancer. Clodronate (dichloromethylene-diphosphonate) has been shown to be effective in palliation of bone pain in prostate cancer when given intravenously in 16 of 17 patients in one study[23], and in 29 of 41 (71%) in another[24]. The only side-effects noted were slight gastrointestinal discomfort when the patients were continued on oral therapy.

Local Radiotherapy

External-beam radiotherapy has been employed for many years as a form of palliation for painful skeletal metastases due to prostate cancer. The probability of effective pain relief is around 70–80% when radiother-

apy is given either as a single dose (8 Gy), or as a short two-week (20 Gy) or three-week (30 Gy) course. When, as is often the case, there are multiple sites of bone pain, local therapy is less effective.

Wide-Field Radiotherapy

Wide-field radiation treatment may sometimes be an option for some patients with intractable pain from widespread metastases. In one collaborative study, hemibody irradiation (6 Gy to upper body and 8 Gy to lower body) resulted in pain-free status being achieved in 30% of patients, partial response in 50%, and no change in 20%. Eighty percent of responses had occurred within 1 week, and the mean duration of pain relief was 3 months. Nausea, vomiting and diarrhoea occurred to mild or moderate extent in 35% of patients. In 15%, however, this was classified as severe or life-threatening. Haematological effects were also classified as severe or life-threatening in 9% of cases[25].

Strontium-89 chloride (Metastron)

The use of the beta-emitting isotope Strontium-89 chloride (Metastron) constitutes a major therapeutic advance for the pain control of patients with prostate cancer. Strontium-89 follows the biological pathways of calcium within the body and decays with a half-life of 50.5 days. Although it is washed out of healthy bone, it localizes preferentially at the sites of increased mineral turnover which characterize osteoblastic metastases. The turnover of Strontium-89 within normal trabecular bone has a half-life of around 14 days, whereas metastatic deposits appear to retain the isotope almost indefinitely.

A number of published trials indicate that Strontium-89 is safe and provides pain relief in up to 78% of patients[26]. For example, in a prospective, randomized study of 32 patients with metastatic cancer using a crossover design against placebo, complete pain relief was only seen after Strontium-89 administration[27]. One recent study showed that it produced a 50% reduction in analgesic requirements in 55% of patients. In the UK Metastron trial 284 patients with painful bone metastases were stratified into two groups according to suitability for local radiotherapy or hemibody (wide-field) irradiation and then randomized within each group to receive either 200 MBq (5.4 mCi) Strontium-89 or the assigned form of external radiotherapy. Pain response at the site of presenting pain was similar in patients treated with either Strontium-89 or external beam radiotherapy, but patients treated with Strontium-89 were less likely to experience new sites of pain. Porter and McEwan[29] have also shown that the isotope delays disease progression and is cost effective by virtue of reduced analgesic and hospitalization costs[30].

Side-effects from Strontium-89 consist mainly of mild haematological toxicity, usually thrombocytopaenia. When this is seen, platelet decreases range from 24–70% and only occasionally meet the criteria for toxicity used to assess cytotoxic chemotherapy. Platelet nadir is dose related and is usually reached 5–7 weeks post-treatment. The leukocyte nadir also occurs around this time, and the effect persists for up to 3 months[31]. As approximately 90% of Strontium-89 is excreted through the kidneys (the remainder undergoing biliary excretion), care should be taken with patients with renal insufficiency. Patients receiving Strontium-89 should also be instructed to dispose of their urine by double flushing since the urine radioactivity, though slight, is measureable.

Patients receiving Strontium-89 should fulfil the following criteria:

- More than one site of skeletal metastasis and diffuse painful sites.
- WBC count >3000/cubic mm and platelet count >60,000/cubic mm.
- Life expectancy >3 months.

- No change in hormonal treatment or chemotherapy within 30 days.

The standard dose is 148 MBq (4 mCi), administered by a slow intravenous injection into a fast running IV line, avoiding extravasation. Pain relief typically occurs in 1–2 weeks and rarely takes 4 weeks or more. If the first injection is not beneficial, the second will probably be no more effective. In the 80% or so of patients who are responsive, the effects of Strontium-89 should last 3 months or longer, after which a further dose may be required.

TERMINAL CARE

Eventually, in spite of all therapeutic efforts, 70% of patients with metastatic prostate cancer will deteriorate and die from their disease, the remainder dying from comorbid conditions. The terminal stages of this illness may be distressing for all concerned because of severe pain from metastatic deposits, and are usually best handled by a team effort involving the relatives, an experienced palliative-care team and the family practitioner. The urologist should be readily available for consultation concerning modifications of therapy and the advisability of eventually transferring the patient to either hospital or preferably a unit specialized in the care of the terminally ill.

REFERENCES

1 Scher HI, Kelly WK. Flutamide withdrawal syndrome: its impact on clinical trials in hormone-refractory prostatic cancer. J Clin Oncol 1993;**11**:1566–1572.

2 Landstrom M, Damber JE, Bergh A. Estrogen treatment postpones the castration-induced dedifferentiation of Dunning R3327-PAP prostatic adenocarcinoma. Prostate 1994;**25 (1)**:10–18.

3 Andersson SB, Gunnarsson PO, Nilsson T, et al. Metabolism of estramustine phosphate (Estracyt) in patients with prostatic carcinoma. European Journal of Drug Metabolism and Pharmacokinetics 1981;**6**:149–154.

4 Stearns ME, Tew KD. Antimicrotubule effects of estramustine, an antiprostatic tumor drug. Canc Res 1985;**45**:3891–3897.

5 Hansenson M, Lundh B, Hartley-Asp B, et al. Growth-inhibiting effect of estramustine on two prostatic carcinoma cell lines, LNCaP and LNCaP-r. Urol Res 1988;**16**:357–361.

6 Hartley-Asp B. Estramustine induced mitotic arrest in two human prostatic cell lines DU 145 and PC–3. Prostate 1984;**5**:93–100.

7 Murphy GP, Slack NH. Response criteria for the prostate of the USA National Prostatic Cancer Project. Prostate 1980;**1**:375–382.

8 Olivier S, Formento ,P, Fischel JL, et al. Epidermal growth factor expression and Suramin cytotoxicity in vitro. Eur J Cancer 1990;**29A**:245–247.

9 Pollak M, Richard M. Suramin blockade of insulin-like growth factor I-stimulated proliferation of osteosarcoma cells. J Natl Cancer Inst 1990;**82**:1349–1352.

10 Pollak M, Polychronakos C, Richard M. Suramin interferes with the binding of insulin-like growth factor I (IGF-I) to IGF-I receptors. Proc Am Assoc Cancer Res 1990;**31**:47–51.

11 Myers C, Cooper M, Stein C, et al. Suramin: a novel growth factor antagonist with activity in hormone-refractory prostate cancer. J Clin Oncol 1992;**10**:881–889.

12 Eisenberger MA, Reyno LM, Jodrell DI. Suramin, an active drug for prostate cancer; interim observations in a phase I trial. J Natl Cancer Inst 1993;**85**:611–621.

13 Rowinsky EK, Onetto N, Canetta RM, et al. Taxol: the first of the taxanes, an important new class of antitumor agents. Sem Urol 1992;**19**:646–662.

14 Stearns ME, Wang M. Taxol blocks processes essential for prostate tumor cell (PC-3 ML) invasion and metastases. *Cancer Res* 1994;**52**:3776–3778.

15 Roth BJ, Yeap BY, Wilding G, *et al.* Taxol in advanced, hormone-refractory carcinoma of the prostate. *Cancer* 1993;**72(8)**:2457–2460.

16 Hudes G, Obasaju C, McAleer C, *et al.* Phase I pharmacologic study of 96-HR infusional Taxol combined with estramustine. *Proc ASCO* 1994;**13**:188-Abst 465.

17 Pienta KJ, Nguyen NM, Lehr JE. Treatment of prostate cancer in the rat with the synthetic retinoid fenretinide. *Canc Res* 1993;**53**:224–226.

18 Dijkman GA, Van Moorselaar RJA, Van Ginckel R, *et al.* Antitumoral effects of liarozole in androgen-dependent and independent R3327-Dunning prostate adenocarcinomas. *J Urol* 1994;**151**:217–222.

19 Seidman AD, Scher HI, Petrylak D, *et al.* Estramustine and vinblastine: use of prostate specific antigen as a clinical trial end point for hormone refractory prostatic cancer. *J Urol* 1992;**147**:931–934.

20 Scher HI, Sternberg C, Heston WDW. Etoposide in prostate cancer: experimental studies and phase II trial in patients with bidimensionally measurable disease. *Cancer Chemother Pharmacol* 1986;**18**:24–26.

21 Pienta KJ, Lehr JE. Inhibition of prostate cancer growth by estramustine and etoposide: evidence for interactions at the nuclear matrix. *J Urol* 1993;**149**:1622–1625.

22 Pienta KJ, Redman BG, Hussain M, *et al.* A combination of estramustine and etoposide orally may be an effective regimen in the treatment of hormone refractory prostate cancer. *Proc Am Soc Clin Oncol* 1993;**12**:246–251.

23 Adami S, Salvagno G, Guarrera G, *et al.* Dichloromethylene-diphosphonate in patients with prostatic carcinoma metastatic to the skeleton. *J Urol* 1985;**134**:1152–1154.

24 Vorreuther R. Biphosphonates as an adjunct to palliative therapy of bone metastases from prostatic carcinoma. A pilot study on clodronate. *Br J Urol* 1993;**72**:792–795.

25 Veronesi A, Zattoni F, Frutaci S, *et al.* Estramustine (Estracyt) treatment of T3-T4 prostatic carcinoma. *Prostate* 1982;**3**:159–164.

26 Crawford ED, Balmer C, Kozlowski JM, *et al.* The use of Strontium-89 for palliation of pain from bone metastases associated with hormone-refractory prostate cancer. *Urology* 1994;**44**:481–485.

27 Lewington V, McEwan AJ, Ackery DM, *et al.* A prospective, randomized double-blind crossover study to examine the efficacy of Strontium-89 in pain palliation in patients with advanced prostate cancer metastatic to bone. *Eur J Cancer* 1991;**27(8)**:954–958.

28 Bolger JJ, Dearnoley DP, Kirk D, *et al.* Strontium-89 (Metastron) versus external beam radiotherapy in patients with painful bone metastases from prostate cancer: preliminary report of a multicentre trial. *Semin Oncol* 1993;**20(Suppl 2)**:32–33.

29 Porter AT, McEwan AJB. Strontium-89 as an adjuvant to external beam irradiation improves pain relief and delays disease progression in advanced prostate cancer: results of a randomized, controlled trial. *Semin Oncol* 1993;**20(Suppl 2)**:38–43.

30 McEwan AJB, Amyotte GA, McGowan DG. A retrospective analysis of the cost-effectiveness of treatment with Metastron (Strontium-89) in patients with prostate cancer metastatic to bone. *Nuc Med Comm* 1994;**15**:499–504.

31 Robinson RG. Strontium-89-precursor targeted therapy for pain relief of blastic metastatic disease. *Cancer* 1993;**72**:3433–3435.

32 Benson RC, Gill GM. Estramustine phosphate compared with diethylstilbestrol. A randomized, double-blind, crossover trial for stage D cancer. *Am J Clinic Oncol* 1986;**9**:341–351.

33 Chisholm GD, O'Donoghue EPN, Kennedy CL. The treatment of oestrogen-escaped carcinoma of the prostate with estramustine phosphate. *Br J Urol* 1977;**49**:717–720.

34 Fosså SD, Miller A. Treatment of advanced carcinoma of the prostate with estramustine phosphate. *J Urol* 1976;**115**:406–408.

35 Jönsson G, Högberg B, Nilsson T. Treatment of advanced prostatic carcinoma with estramustine phosphate. *Scan J Urol Nephrol* 1977;**11**:231–238.

36 Küss R, Khoury S, Richard F, *et al.* Estramustine phosphate in the treatment of advanced prostatic cancer. *Br J Urol* 1980;**52**:29–33.

37 Leistenschneider W, Nagel R. Estracyt therapy of advanced prostatic cancer with special reference to control of therapy with cytology and DNA cytophotometry. *Eur Urol* 1980;**6**:111–115.

38 Lindberg B. Treatment of rapidly progressing prostatic carcinoma with Estracyt. *J Urol* 1972;**108**:303–306.

39 Mittelman A, Shukla SK, Murphy GP. Extended therapy of stage D carcinoma of the prostate with oral Estracyt. *J Urol* 1976;**115**:409–412.

40 Murphy GP, Gibbons RP, Johanson DE, *et al.* A comparison of estramustine phosphate and streptozotocin in patients with advanced prostatic carcinoma who have had extensive radiation. *J Urol* 1977;**118**:288–291.

41 Soloway MS, de Kernion JB, Gibbons RP, *et al.* Comparison of estramustine phosphate and vincristine alone or in combination for patients with advanced hormone refractory previously irradiated carcinoma of the prostate. *J Urol* 1981;**125**:664–667.

42 Soloway MS, Beckley S, Brady MF, *et al.* A comparison of estramustine phosphate versus cisplatinum alone versus estramustine phosphate plus cisplatinum in patients with advanced hormone refractory cancer who have had extensive irradiation to the pelvis or lumbosacral area. *J Urol* 1983;**129**:56–61.

43 Eisenberger M, Simon R, O'Dwyer P, *et al.* A re-evaluation of non-hormonal cytotoxic chemotherapy in the treatment of prostatic carcinoma. *J Clin Oncol* 1985;**3**:827–841.

44 Scott WW, Gibbons RP, Johnson DE, *et al..* The continued evaluation of the effects of chemotherapy in patients with advanced carcinoma of the prostate. *J Urol* 1976;**116**:211–213.

45 Murphy GP, Gibbons RP, Johnson DE, *et al.* A comparison of estramustine phosphate and streptozotocin in patients with prostatic carcinoma who had extensive irradiation. *J Urol* 1977;**118**:288–291.

46 Schmidt JD, Scott WW, Gibbons RP, *et al.*. Comparison of procarbazine, imidazole-carbamide and cyclophosphamide in relapsing patients with advanced carcinoma of the prostate. J Urol 1979;**121**:185–189.

47 Loening SA, Scott WW, de Kernion JB, *et al.* A comparison of hydroxyurea, methyl-chlorohexyl-nitrosourea and cyclophosphamide in patients with advanced prostate cancer. J Urol 1981;**125**:812–816.

48 Soloway MS, de Kernion JB, Gibbons RP, *et al.* Comparison of estramustine phosphate and vincristine alone or in combination for patients with advanced hormone refractory previously irradiated carcinoma of the prostate. J Urol 1981;**125**:664–667.

49 Soloway M, Beckley S, Brady MF, *et al.* A comparison of estramustine phosphate, versus cis-platinum alone versus estramustine phosphate plus cis-platinum in patients with advanced hormone refractory prostate cancer who had extensive irradiation to the pelvis or lumbosacral area. J Urol 1983;**129**:56–61.

50 Oesterling JE, Jacobsen SJ, Chute CG, *et al.* Serum PSA in a community-based population of healthy men. JAMA. 1993;**270**:860–864.

CHAPTER 14

REASONS TO BE CHEERFUL

Although at first sight the statistics may seem depressing, there are in fact many reasons to feel increasingly optimistic about the prospects for sufferers of prostate cancer.

EARLIER DETECTION

Awareness about prostate cancer, among both the general public and health-care professionals, has risen steeply over the past few years: a 'Cinderella subject' up to the 1980s, prostatic diseases have recently become a favourite topic of conversation of men over 50 as well as their wives and families. In the USA and Europe, the media have developed an almost obsessive interest in the subject, and this fixation, which has already resulted in increased health-care seeking behaviour by men beyond middle age, is now being translated into earlier clinical detection in clinical practice – the 'stage migration' so frequently emphasized in previous chapters. However, while this potentially provides the means of achieving cure in many more patients, the possibility of over-treatment of men whose cancers were destined never to become clinically significant still remains a matter of some concern.

BETTER FUNDING FOR RESEARCH

New-found public interest in prostate cancer has also resulted in a recent increase in spending on clinical research, although this remains only a small proportion of the funds directed towards other major cancer killers, such as breast, lung and colonic carcinoma. The traditional explanation for the parsimony of governmental and research-body funding for prostate cancer has been the unimpressive number of average life years – around nine – lost due to the disease. However, as pointed out in Chapter 2, as the disease is so com-

mon, the cumulative loss of life years due to prostate cancer is third among all cancers; those nine twilight years at jeopardy in the later decades of life are also often considered *the* most precious by both the patients and their loved ones, and now the more elderly segment of society is becoming more vocal about its right to medical care.

The increased awareness surrounding the clinical aspects of prostate cancer has also resulted in an increase in funding for basic research which is now yielding significant rewards. The disease area has attracted the attention of experts other than urologists, and many more players have recently become involved – family practitioners, biostatisticians, epidemiologists, health economy and policy analysts all now contribute expertise and opinions. Although their views may sometimes be difficult to integrate with those of urologists – the group who predominantly provide actual care to the patients – new perspectives on cost:benefit ratios of various treatment options and economic modelling can only enhance our understanding of the socio-economic impact of this very prevalent disease.

The trend towards detection of earlier stage prostate cancer in the USA has become most marked since 1987, the year when widespread PSA testing became available. Since then, there has been a rapid rise in the number of transrectal biopsies undertaken (**14.1**), and therefore a rise in the number of potentially curable prostate cancers diagnosed, as well as the number of curative procedures performed (**14.2**), such as radical prostatectomies. The question remains open as to whether all of this activity will eventually translate into a reduction in the overall mortality of prostate cancer, but patients with metastatic disease are already reputed to be becoming less common in everyday urological practice, at least in the USA.

MORE ACCURATE DIAGNOSIS

While PSA staging carries indisputable potential for the earlier diagnosis of prostate cancer, it also carries the drawback of a significant incidence of false positive results. Since transrectal ultrasound imaging does not reliably identify every small focus of cancer, effectively every individual testing positive (PSA >4.0 ng/ml) will require transrectal ultrasound-guided biopsy to rule out cancer. Around 15% of screened populations of men over 50 years test PSA-positive, but only 2–5% prove positive in fact on biopsy. Thus, between two-thirds and four-fifths of men will be worried that they *may* have cancer until the biopsy result is known (the psychological effects and sequelae of this period of anxiety are unknown), and around 3% of those testing false positive and undergoing biopsy will suffer significant morbidity from the procedure (such as sepsis or bleeding). However, the near future holds the promise of more specific PSA tests. New assays are currently under development, based on differentiating free-PSA from complexed-PSA, and should significantly reduce the incidence of false positive testing[1].

Since serum PSA levels show a tendency to rise with age, a given individual screened by PSA testing will be more likely to test positive simply by virtue of being older. While the incidence of prostate cancer also rises steeply with age, it is probably more important to diagnose the disease in younger men because their greater life expectancy gives them more years 'at risk' of developing disease progression and metastases. These considerations have led Oesterling *et al.*[2] to advocate age-adjustment of PSA cut-offs (**Table 14.1**) based on the 95-percentile values for PSA in a population of men *without* prostate cancer.

Another promising avenue is the extra information available from sequential PSA determinations – or the so-called 'PSA slope'. Carter *et al.* compared serial PSA values in individuals with BPH, prostate cancer and controls, and reported that an annualized PSA rise of more than 0.75 ng/ml was associated with a diagnosis of cancer (**14.3**). In his ongoing study of PSA screening, Brawer[3] reported a diagnosis of prostate cancer in 17% of those men whose PSA increased by more than 20% over one year. Further data are currently accumulating on the diagnostic value of sequential PSA measurement.

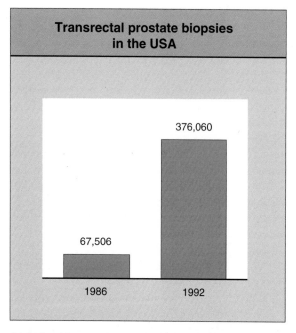

14.1 The rising number of TRUS-guided biopsies in the USA between 1986 and 1992. (Medicare data kindly supplied by L Holtgrewe.)

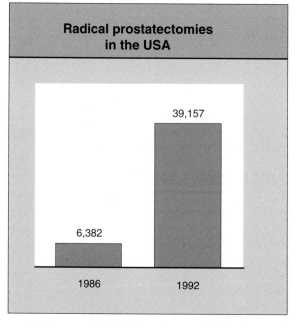

14.2 The rising number of radical prostatectomies performed in the USA. (Medicare data kindly supplied by L Holtgrewe.)

ENHANCED PROGNOSTIC INDICATORS

As previously emphasized, the central issue in prostate cancer management is deciding clinically which lesions should be managed conservatively, and which more aggressively. Although Gleason scoring and tumour-volume estimation give a reasonable indication of subsequent tumour behaviour, molecular biological markers seem to hold the promise of more accurate prognostic information. Already, E-cadherin estimation seems to correlate with subsequent metastatic potential[4], and a host of other markers (see Chapter 2) are currently being intensively evaluated in this context. It appears to be only a matter of time before we will be in a position to prognosticate the future behaviour of a given prostate cancer much more accurately, and thereby balance the risks of tumour progression against the probabilities of demise due to other comorbid conditions, before advising a specific form of therapy.

Evolving molecular biological techniques should also permit the identification of those individuals at particular risk of prostate cancer because of a familial tendency. Linkage analysis on the chromosomal configurations of groups of individuals with a strong fam-

ily history of prostate cancer should soon result in the identification of a 'prostate cancer gene', analogous to the 'breast cancer gene' already characterized[5]. Individuals carrying this gene (or more plausibly suffering from a particular tumour-suppressor gene deletion) would be obvious candidates for close surveillance, early biopsy and therapy before extracapsular extension and metastatic progression occur.

Better Staging

One of the more potent arguments against the use of radical prostatectomy for the management of localized prostate cancer has been the historically high (30–40%) positive margin rate. These patients are at high risk of subsequent disease recurrence and would, in most cases, probably be better managed by alternative, less invasive, forms of therapy. New imaging technology, employing endorectal MRI coils as well as developments such as radioisotopes attached to prostate cancer-seeking compounds, now hold the prospect of more accurate tumour volume estimation and staging information. This should eventually translate into better patient selection for curative procedures.

Table 14.1 Age-specific reference ranges for PSA as suggested by Oesterling	
Age (years)	Upper limit of serum PSA (ng/ml)
40–49	2.5
50–59	3.5
60–69	4.5
70–79	6.5

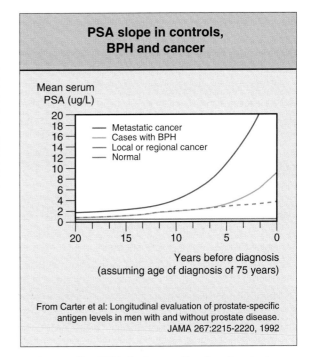

14.3 Annualized PSA rise in a small series of controls, patients with BPH and those with prostate cancer.

Identification of Micrometastases with Polymerase Chain Reaction Technology

Currently, one of the greatest drawbacks in accurately staging prostate cancer is the inability to detect the prevalence of systemic micrometastases. It is not until metastases reach a certain critical size that they can be identified with imaging such as radionuclide bone scanning. This being the case, a number of patients are treated for disease that is assumed to be localized at a stage when, in fact, micrometastases have occurred and more systemic forms of therapy are appropriate. The recent advent of polymerase chain reaction (PCR) technology have provided the means whereby these micrometastases can be identified.

PCR technology allows the amplification of tiny amounts of either DNA or RNA. In the normal individual, transcription of the portion of the DNA that encodes prostate specific antigen for messenger RNA, and subsequently PSA, should be confined to epithelial cells of the prostate. The finding, therefore, of tiny amounts of mRNA for PSA either in the blood stream or in bone marrow aspirate would be highly suggestive of the presence of micrometastases of prostate-cancer tumour cells.

The technology of the polymerase chain reaction is illustrated in **14.4**. Briefly, double-stranded complementary DNA (cDNA) is made from the mRNA of the sample by using random primers. Primers specific to the upper and lower strands of the cDNA to be amplified are added to a reaction mixture, and a thermostable DNA polymerase (originally isolated from the bacterium *Thermus aquaticus*, which thrives naturally in the water of hot springs in a temperature of 75°C) is added to cause transcription of the specific complimentary DNA sequence for PSA. This procedure is repeated between 30 and 35 times to increase exponentially the amount of cDNA between the two primers. This amplification process allows the detection of one abnormal cell from a population of between 10^6 and 10^7, provided that the abnormal cell produces a unique mRNA sequence. Reverse transcriptase PCR technology was originally used to detect the bcr/abl mRNA produced by chronic myelogenous leukaemia (CML) cells. The reverse transcriptase PCR of bone marrow aspirates could identify residual disease in CML, despite an apparently complete response to chemotherapy[6]. Because prostate cancer produces a unique protein, PSA, and spreads primarily to bone marrow, which is accessible before definitive therapy is undertaken, it is in many ways an ideal tumour model for identifying micrometastases.

To detect micrometastatic disease in patients with prostate cancer, PSA mRNA has been amplified by Wood *et al.*[7], and sensitivity and specificity experiments using PSA-specific primers performed. No PSA mRNA was identified in peripheral blood mononuclear or

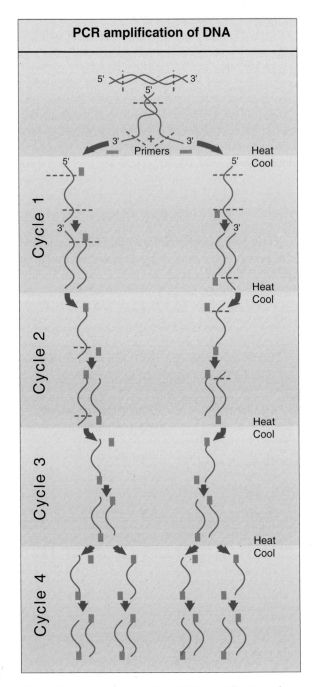

14.4 Polymerase chain reaction (PCR) amplification of a DNA segment can be used to detect PSA producing cells outside the prostate.

bone marrow cells in healthy volunteers, but sensitivity experiments using LNCaP human prostate-cancer cell line mixed with bone-marrow cells were carried out which were able to identify one LNCaP cell from a population of 10^6 bone marrow cells. These results suggested that the test might be clinically valuable.

Subsequently, Wood et al.[7] performed a small study on patients suffering from prostate cancer. Two patients had known metastatic disease as demonstrated by a positive bone scan, and five had clinically localized disease. Both patients with known metastases showed up positive on the test. One of the five patients who had clinically localized disease was also positive and this patient's tumour extended to the surgical margins of resection at radical prostatectomy.

Recently, the Columbia University Group[8] have used similar molecular based technology using peripheral blood instead of bone marrow cells to identify the presence of micrometastases in patients suffering from prostate cancer. In a sizeable control group, all of the patients had negative PCR results for PSA. By contrast, of the 20 patients with metastatic prostate cancer, 16 (80%) had positive reactions. In a group of 80 patients with various stages of clinically localized disease, the PSA PCR test had a 67% sensitivity for detecting capsular penetration and 87% sensitivity for detecting disease at the surgical margin as well as an 83% sensitivity for detecting seminal vesical invasion. By contrast, a similar assay for prostate specific membrane antigen (PSMA) did not appear to correlate nearly as well with either the presence of metastases or the pathological stage of localized prostate cancer.

PROSPECTS FOR IMPROVED THERAPY

The treatment options for patients with prostate cancer will undoubtedly continue to expand and improve. In expert hands, the incontinence rate within 6 months of radical prostatectomy should now be less than 3%, potency may be preserved at least in younger men, and post-operative mortality should be exceedingly uncommon. Technical improvements in surgical technique – for example, with the development of an automatic anastomotic 'gun' or other devices to facilitate surgery – could conceivably reduce the incontinence rate to virtually zero. A recent series of 3170 radical prostatectomies from the Mayo Clinic reported a mortality rate of only 0.3%[9].

Radiotherapy for prostate cancer is also likely to become more effective. Conformational techniques already permit better localization of tumoricidal doses to the prostate, thus reducing morbidity due to the involvement of adjacent structures (**14.5**)[10]. Early reports suggest that development of new modalities of radiation therapy, such as fast-neutron treatment generated using cyclotron technology, may enhance tumoricidal activity without significantly increasing side-effects[11].

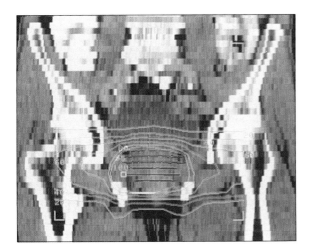
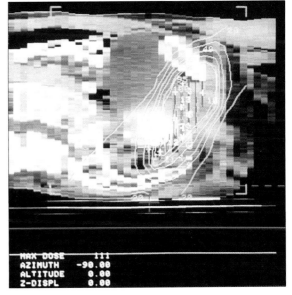

14.5 Conformal imaging of the prostate prior to cyclotron treatment using accelerated neutrons
a. AP view.
b. Lateral view.

Pharmacotherapy

Many of the potential therapeutic advances that offer the best prospects for future sufferers of prostate cancer are pharmacological. As already discussed, maximal androgen blockade seems, at least in a subset of patients, to hold a small but significant advantage over monotherapy with LHRH analogues. The recent data relating to Casodex, an antiandrogen, suggest that this compound, when administered orally at a dose of 150 mg once per day, may be at least as efficacious as conventional therapy, but without the quality of life impairment due to adverse effects on sexual function. There may also be a role for antiandrogen therapy in earlier stage, localized disease, especially in older patients, but this needs to be confirmed by long-term, randomized studies.

Chemoprevention

Chemoprevention can be defined as the administration of drugs with the aim of interfering with carcinogenesis, cancer growth or tumour progression. In the context of carcinoma of the prostate, where latent microscopic cancer is so common, the most likely target for chemoprevention would probably be the inhibition of steps that are critical to cancer progression. Men between 40 and 70 years of age might be suitable for such intervention if it were to become available. If the toxicity of the interventional drug were minimal, potentially it could be offered to all men older than 40 years in areas where prostate cancer is common. Alternatively, if the drug toxicity was relatively minor, but still present, and if better markers of prostate cancer progression were developed, the middle-aged population could be screened with a view to inclusion only of those at high risk of cancer development and progression. Chemoprevention is clearly likely to be of little or no benefit in men older than 70 years of age.

Characteristics of available chemopreventive drugs

The list of potential chemopreventive agents is long. It appears that, based on pre-clinical studies as well as on chemoprevention studies in other human tumours, four categories of drugs might be considered for prostate cancer chemoprevention (**Table 14.2**).

Difluoromethylornithine (DFMO)

DFMO is an effective chemopreventive agent in a variety of animal tumours by virtue of its activity as an irreversible inhibitor of ornithine decarboxylase, the enzyme responsible for the first and rate-limiting step in mammalian polyamine synthesis. Polyamines are normal cell constituents that are important for the regulation of cell proliferation and cell differentiation; the mammalian prostate contains some of the highest concentrations of polyamines anywhere in the body. The administration of DFMO to immature animals prevents normal prostatic development. It has been shown that DFMO inhibits ornithine decarboxylase activity in the Dunning R3327 rat prostatic carcinoma, and also inhibits the growth of this tumour both *in vitro* and *in vivo*. In animal studies, a cyclic regimen of administration involving low doses of the drug reduced toxicity while maintaining chemotherapeutic efficacy. As such, DFMO seems to deserve serious consideration in prostate cancer chemoprevention[12].

Retinoids

Vitamin A (retinol) and its natural analogues (retinoids) are important modulators of epithelial proliferation and differentiation (**14.6**). Retinoids appear to exert their activity by binding to specific nuclear receptors. Mice that had these receptors eliminated by sophisticated gene deletion techniques were born with a dysplastic or absent prostate gland, thus establishing an important potential role for retinoids in prostate development. Many studies have demonstrated the ability of retinoids to suppress carcinogenesis, both *in vitro* and *in vivo*, and synthetic retinoids were shown to inhibit the growth of a carcinogen-induced prostate cancer, perhaps by enhancing the expression of transforming growth factor beta (TGF beta)[13]. The synthetic retinoid, fenretinide, when added to the diet, reduced the incidence and slowed the progression of oncogene-induced prostate cancer in mice[14]. Whereas epidemiological studies attempting to correlate dietary retinoids with a risk of developing prostate cancers have usually been equivocal, evidence that low serum retinol levels correlate with an increased risk of prostate cancer is somewhat stronger[15,16].

The natural retinoids, although effective in inhibiting carcinogenesis, display significant toxicities which preclude their use as general chemopreventive agents. Synthetic retinoid analogues that retain their biological activity and possess a favourable toxicity profile are, however, currently available. The best known, and most extensively studied, is fenretinide. The safety of fenretinide has been demonstrated in a large breast-cancer chemoprevention trial in Europe, which involved the administration of a daily dose of 200 mg, with a three-day period each month when the drug was not given[17]. Several groups in the USA are currently planning chemoprevention prostate cancer studies using this compound.

Finasteride

The prostate is dependent upon dihydrotestosterone (DHT) for its development and subsequent function. The ability of drugs like finasteride to suppress DHT levels without significantly altering testosterone-dependent functions like muscle strength and libido, has prompted the US National Cancer Institute to propose a large chemopreventive study using this agent. This study, which has now begun accrual, aims to enrol 1800 healthy men between 55 and 70 years of age who will be randomized into treatment groups receiving either 5 mg of oral finasteride each day or placebo. Both groups will be biopsied at the end of 7 years and followed for an overall period of at least 10 years. The study's design will allow detection of a 25% decrease in new tumours or local progression with a roughly 90% statistical certainty.

Vitamin D

Recently, Schwartz and his colleagues proposed that low levels of vitamin D could increase the risk of clinical prostate cancer, and they presented some epidemiological evidence to support this theory[18]. Experimental evidence also suggests that vitamin D does possess tumour-inhibitory properties. The human prostate and prostate cancer cell lines contain vitamin D receptors and, furthermore, vitamin D can promote differentiation of prostate cancer lines *in vitro*. Administration of high doses of vitamin D is, however, associated with toxicity including hypercalcaemia. Analogues of vitamin D that do not induce hypercalcaemia have now been synthesized, and might be considered for evaluation in prostate cancer chemoprevention.

Potential for Gene Therapy

Recently there has been a veritable explosion in interest in the concept of gene therapy for many neoplastic and non-neoplastic disease areas, and some of these developments may have special application to prostate cancer. Gene therapy involves the transference of new genetic material into the cells of a patient in the prospect of therapeutic benefit, hopefully with the induction of few concomitant side effects. In order for gene therapy to work it will of course be necessary to select a gene which encodes the desired therapeutic effect and secondly to develop effective vectors for gene delivery[19,20]. In essence, gene therapy offers three potential mechanisms by which patients with prostatic cancer may be helped:

- Restoration of normal controls over cell division. This could be conceivably achieved by reintroducing deleted tumour suppressor genes or alternatively by insertion of functional homologues which inhibit prostate tumour oncogene expression.
- By enhancement of the natural host cytotoxic and immunostimulatory defence mechanisms against cancer[21].
- Either the delivery of toxic products specifically to cancer cells or the induction of sensitivity to toxic drugs which specifically kill prostate cancer cells.

Table 14.2 Potential chemopreventive agents
Difluoromethylornithine (DFMO)
Fenretinide (N-4-hydroxyphenyl retinamide) and other retinoids
Finasteride (5-alpha reductase inhibitor)
Vitamin D analogues

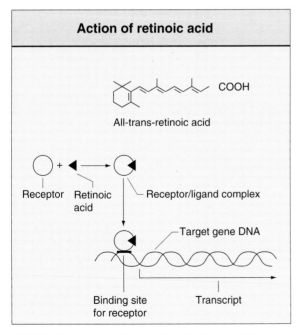

Action of retinoic acid

COOH

All-trans-retinoic acid

Receptor   Retinoic acid   Receptor/ligand complex

Target gene DNA

Binding site for receptor   Transcript

14.6 Mechanism of action of retinoids in modulating gene expression.

Effector genes and their mechanisms

As discussed in Chapter 3, prostatic cell division is regulated by a delicate balance of growth promoting oncogenes and growth constraining tumour suppressor genes. Loss of tumour suppressor gene activity may remove a constraint on oncogene expression and thereby allow prostate cancer cells to proliferate. One potential for gene therapy therefore is to facilitate reinsertion of negative regulatory sequences. The genetic insertion of wild-type tumour suppressor genes could prevent neoplastic cell behaviour and restore normal growth patterns[23].

Cytokines

Among the most important elements of anti-tumour activity in normal individuals are naturally occurring cytokines. These substances are able to induce direct tumoricidal effects and they are also capable of initiating and maintaining natural immune surveillance against cancer. Cytokine genes could be transferred into either tumour cells or natural effector cells, thereby promoting an immune attack against neoplastic tissue and subsequent immune surveillance[24].

Cytoreductive therapy

Currently, much interest is focused on the transference of drug susceptibility by gene therapy. After transfer of a gene to cancer cells encoding an enzyme which converts a prodrug into a suicide substrate, the prodrug could be administered systemically thereby eliminating malignant target cells that have been genetically modified. This approach has been pioneered as brachytherapy in malignant brain tumours. One therapeutic combination is intravenous ganciclovir administration after herpes simplex virus thymidine kinase (HSV-tk) gene transfer. In this system, HSV-tk phosphorylation of ganciclovir (GCV) leads to the formation of ganciclovir triphosphate, a potent nucleotide competitor which interferes with DNA synthesis and thereby results in programmed cell death.

Gene Delivery Techniques

Integral to all forms of gene therapy is the vector used for gene transfer. Vectors are usually engineered DNA or RNA sequences which contain a site into which a therapeutic gene can be inserted. These vectors are then used to transfer the therapeutic gene into target cancer cells. The therapeutic gene in question is positioned in the vector adjacent to a promoter sequence for RNA polymerase which allows for the expression of messenger RNA of this gene after the vector enters the target for gene therapy. Promoter sequences control the expression of downstream genes and thus constitute a critical engineering component of most gene transfer vectors.

Retrovirus transduction

Genetic material in retroviruses occurs in the form of double-stranded RNA. Once an individual cell is infected with a retrovirus, the RNA genome is reverse transcribed into DNA which then stably integrates into the host DNA. Although retroviral vector mediated gene transfer can be durable, the decay of the viral titre when given intravenously will often impede their potential for direct intravenous *in vivo* gene transfer to disease cells. In fact, retroviruses appear far better suited for *in vitro* gene transfer into living cells that are subsequently returned to the patient (**14.7**). Unfortunately retroviral vectors require target cell proliferation for genomic integration; since gene transfer will only succeed in actively dividing cells. In addition, the possibility of pathogenic metagenesis during chromosomal insertion of the vector and the difficulty in isolating high enough titres for clinical use are further limitations associated with this vector system.

Adenovirus transduction

Unlike retroviruses, adenoviruses are capable of infecting non-dividing cells and can also potentially carry large quantities of genetic material. They are therefore capable of mediating durable genetic transduction and

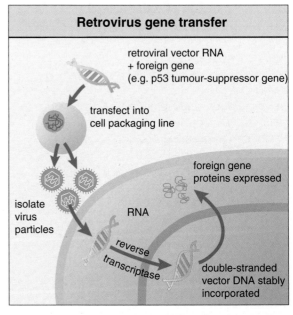

Retrovirus gene transfer

retroviral vector RNA
+ foreign gene
(e.g. p53 tumour-suppressor gene)

transfect into
cell packaging line

isolate
virus
particles

foreign gene
proteins expressed

RNA

reverse
transcriptase

double-stranded
vector DNA stably
incorporated

14.7 Retroviruses can be used to stably transfer genetic material into host cells.

are themselves sufficiently stable for potential direct *in vivo* gene transfer. However, integration of adenovirus genomes into target cell DNA has so far been associated with a greater tendency towards unwanted deletions and rearrangements during gene transfer.

An adenoviral vector none the less has been used to transfect prostate cancer cells with an efficacy as high as 65%[24]; the transfection is of only transient duration however and therefore repeated inoculations may be needed for continuous *in vivo* effective gene delivery. None the less, expression appears to last for up to two weeks and this may be sufficient for adequate immunostimulation. Adeno-associated viruses (AAV) integrate into non dividing cells with a high efficiency but can only accept relatively small fragments of DNA. There is evidence that the AAV genome reproducibly integrates into a region of the human chromosome 19, which in itself has some advantages in terms of manipulation and exploitation. Adenovirus vectors have been chosen for the transmembrane regulatory gene transduction in cystic fibrosis gene therapy, partly because the virus particles are amenable to purification and concentration without significant loss of transduction activity.

However, the sophisticated mechanisms of pathogenicity of the parent viruses from which all of these vectors are derived do require equally sophisticated genetic engineering to render them clinically safe. Currently no single vector possesses all the desirable features for every therapeutic application. Desirable features include permanence of transduction, high efficiency of gene transfer, target tissue specificity and fidelity of gene expressions over time. When choosing a vector system for clinical application, the relative importance of each feature needs to be considered. In a related technique, liposomes can be complexed with effector gene DNA and then injected into the peripheral circulation. Liposomes with target cell membranes can thereby deliver DNA to their cytoplasm. A liposome-DNA complex containing interleukin-2 bearing adeno-associated virus (AAV) has been successfully used by Vieweg *et al* to transfect prostate cancer cells[25] with a roughly 50% efficacy and a stable expression for around 2 weeks duration.

Potential Approaches for Gene Therapy in Prostate Cancer
Restoration of normal growth regulation
As has already been discussed, oncogene activity via specific growth factors and their receptors may well be an important mechanism in the development of the various stages of prostate cancer. In theory, at least, gene therapy could be used to insert functional homologues into existing prostate cancer cells that might inhibit the deleterious effects of abnormal oncogene expression.

Mutations in the tumour suppression gene P53 are known to be associated with uncontrolled proliferation of tumour cells and deletions involving this gene may well be involved in the development of androgen dependent and independent growth of prostate cancer.

In vitro tumour inhibition has been demonstrated in prostate cancer cells in culture by replacing P53 suppressor gene activity which adds credence to the suggestion that mutation and deletion of the P53 tumour suppressor gene may increase malignant potential in this disease[26].

Other tumour suppressor genes including the retinoblastoma (RB gene) may also be important in the development of prostate cancer. Potentially, therefore gene therapy could replace mutated RB genes. *In vitro* studies by Stiener *et al*[27] suggest that the replacement of the RB gene may increase the sensitivity of cells to transforming growth factor beta (TGF beta) and thereby slow tumour growth. Another approach may be to restore androgen receptor activity which potentially could result in the restoration of androgen sensitivity to tumour cells[28].

A number of further growth factors and cell adhesion molecules that can modulate prostate cancer cells have been identified, including fibroblast growth factor and transforming growth factors alpha and beta. Currently several groups are studying the oncogenic effects of these specific elements and the ways in which these can be manipulated to facilitate the development of gene therapy. As mentioned earlier in this book, an absence of E-cadherin may be important in the development of metastatic prostatic malignancy[4]; its restoration by gene therapy may potentially be beneficial. The way in which this rapidly evolving knowledge in this field can be clinically utilized for the development of gene therapy for prostate cancer has yet to be fully established, but clearly the potential is enormous.

Cytoreductive Immunotherapy
The most extensively studied form of cytoreductive gene therapy involves augmentation of host immune responses against malignancy by vaccinating affected patients with genetically modified tumour cells. The goal of immunotherapy is to sensitize immune effector cells to tumour antigen, and thereby precipitate a cytotoxic response directed at the tumour with mini-

mal associated systemic toxicity. Recent work in several centres has demonstrated that immunogenicity of neoplastic prostate tissue and its potential susceptibility to immunotherapy[22,23]. Current interest is focused on cytokines and the many growth factors which are involved in the proliferation of both neoplastic cells and cytotoxic cells directed against tumour antigens. A variety of cytokines that modulate antitumour immune response have been used in gene modified tumour vaccines for gene therapy. One of the first studies using this strategy showed induction of anti-tumour effect in nude mice by means of vaccination of tumour cells transduced to secrete interleukin-2 (IL-2). This study aimed to achieve nonspecific (T-cell independent) antitumour effect by producing significant systemic levels of IL-2. Subsequently other cytokines including IL-4, IL-6 and granulocyte-macrophage colony-stimulating factor (GM-CSF), were also shown to have the ability to eliminate microscopic tumour cell deposits when mouse tumour cells were transduced with the respective cytokine genes and when these cytokine-secreting tumours were reintroduced into the animals.

Tumour Vaccines

At present, most tumour vaccine protocols exploit the ability of cytokines to increase tumour cell immunogenicity thereby increasing host cell immune surveillance and tumourlysis. The need for individual patient cancer cell harvesting for cell culture and tumour burden reduction currently make urological surgery a necessary component. After removal of the patient's primary lesion, tumour cells can be cultured and transfected with cytokine genes ex vivo. These cells, with enhanced cytokine production potential, are then readministered to the patient subcutaneously to stimulate an antitumour immune response. Although cytokine production will only occur at the implant site, the stimulated immune effector agents then diffuse throughout the host to pursue and destroy diffuse tumour foci (**14.8**). Studies in animals with subcutaneously inoculated vaccines demonstrate potent specific and long lasting anti-tumour immunity. A tumour vaccine has been recently created in the Dunning R3327 - MatLyLu prostate tumour cell line. Vieweg *et al*[25] investigated an interleukin-2 secreting tumour vaccine which they found could cure animals with established tumour and induce immunological memory in the subjects protecting them from succeeding tumour challenge.

Transfer of Drug Susceptibility Genes

Another form of cytoreductive gene therapy under development involves the transfer of drug susceptibility genes. After transfer of a gene to cancer cells encoding an enzyme which converts a prodrug into a suicide substrain, the prodrug can be administered systemically thereby eliminating malignant target cells that have been genetically modified. Eastham *et al*.[29] have recently used a recombinant adenovirus carrying the herpes simplex virus thymidine kinase (HSV-tk) gene to confer sensitivity to gangciclovir (GCV) to prostate cancer cells in culture.

The 'Bystander Effect'

An important new concept in gene therapy is that of the 'bystander effect'. This refers to the successful destruction of an entire tumour burden despite subtotal transfection of tumour cells with the target gene. This implies some mechanism whereby non-transduced cancer cells in the vicinity of a transduced cancer cell can also be killed after exposure to the drug. The pathways of cell death in the bystander effect still needs elucidation. Clearly there is a risk that this effect could also lead to toxicity related to the bystander effect harming local normal cells in the vicinity of the tumour.

The bystander effect is an important concept in terms of gene therapy for prostate cancer. Prostate tumour masses are known to consist of a very heterogenous collection of cells, some of which are very immature. A sufficiently intense local immune response however, may be enough to ensure that not only mature but also surrounding immature cancer cells will also be destroyed.

Target Tissue Specific Gene Delivery

Vectors are currently being constructed that contain tissue specific promoters which restrict expression of a transferred cytotoxic gene. Prostate cancer is potentially an optimal target for such approaches. By designing a construct with a gene of interest whose expression is controlled by the PSA promoter and regulatory sequences, only cells which normally express PSA will express the transferred therapeutic gene product. Pilot studies have examined this approach by evaluating expression of luciferase (a reporter gene which encodes a readily assayed gene product) transcribed downstream from the human PSA promoter sequence after transfection with prostate cancer cells *in vitro*[24]. Peng *et al*[30] have confirmed the specificity to prostate derived tissue with this approach and increased the activity fourfold by combining the PSA promoter with an upstream cytomegalovirus (CMV) promoter sequence.

In conclusion, the prospects for gene therapy in prostate cancer seem exceedingly promising. For further information the reader is directed to the excellent review by Sander and Simmonds[22] together with that of Sokolov and Belldegrun[31].

CONCLUSION

Some may find the many uncertainties associated with prostate cancer, the most enigmatic of diseases, unsettling. But, as we have tried to convey throughout this book, there are currently numerous grounds for optimism. Although prostate cancer research has lagged behind that of breast cancer – its endocrine-related equivalent in females – this balance is now beginning to be redressed; many of the fundamental issues are currently being tackled in well designed, long-term, randomized studies.

Chemoprevention, screening, and optimal therapy for both localized and metastatic disease are all currently under intense scrutiny. Commercial considerations related to the demographic shift and the rising prevalence of prostate cancer will ensure that the already considerable investment in new pharmacological, molecular, biological and technological therapy continues. Many of the controversies surrounding prostate cancer will be resolved only when the results of long-term, randomized studies are available, but in the meantime it falls to us as clinicians to communicate clearly and sympathetically to our patients and their families the range of diagnostic and treatment options available, together with their various merits and demerits.

As in many other areas of medicine, there are no absolute rights and wrongs in the treatment of prostate cancer; the selection of therapy continues to be often more of an art than a science. Until definitive data are available, we must continue to do the best we can for our patients, even if we do not know all of the answers. It should be remembered that communication with a sympathetic professional, conversant with the very latest information can do as much for the quality of life of the patient as the actual treatment employed.

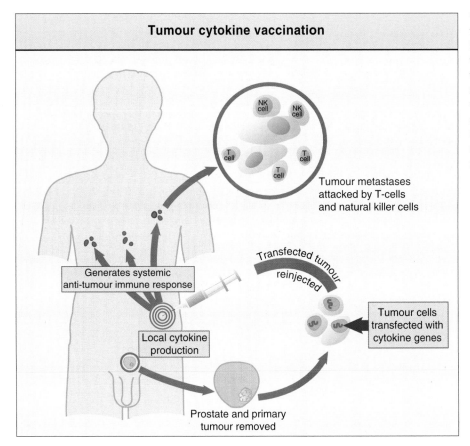

Tumour cytokine vaccination

NK cell
NK cell
T cell
T cell
T cell

Tumour metastases attacked by T-cells and natural killer cells

Transfected tumour reinjected

Tumour cells transfected with cytokine genes

Generates systemic anti-tumour immune response

Local cytokine production

Prostate and primary tumour removed

14.8 Vaccination therapy for prostate cancer may involve harvesting tumour cells, transfecting them with cytokine genes and reintroducing them where they may stimulate immune responses against tumour cells by T cells and natural killer (NK) cells.

REFERENCES

1   Christensson A, Bjork T, Nilsson O, *et al.* Serum prostate specific antigen complexed to alpha-1-antichymotrypsin as an indicator of prostate cancer. J Urol 1993;**150**:100–105.

2   Oesterling JE, Jacobsen SJ, Chute CG, *et al.* The establishment of age-specific reference ranges for prostate-specific antigen. J Urol 1993;**149**:510A.

3   Brawer MK, Beatie J, Wener MH, *et al.* Screening for prostatic carcinoma with prostate specific antigen: results of the second year. J Urol 1993;**150**:106–109.

4   Umbas R, Schalken JA, Aalders TW, *et al.* Expression of cellular adhesion molecule E-cadherin is reduced or absent in high-grade prostate cancer. *Canc Res* 1992;**52**:5104–5109.

5   Black DM, Nicolai H, Borrow J, *et al.* A somatic cell hybrid map of the long arm of human chromosome 17, containing the familial breast cancer locus (BRCA1). *Am J Hum Genetics* 1993;**52(4)**:702–710.

6   Roth MS, Antin JH, Ashe R. Prognostic significance of Philadelphia chromosome positive cells detected by the polymerase chain reaction after allogeneic bone marrow transplant for chronic myelogenous leukaemia. *Blood*, 1992;**79**:276–282.

7   Wood DP, Banks ER, Humphreys S, *et al.* Sensitivity of immunohistochemistry and polymerase chain reaction in deleting prostate cancer cells in bone marrow. J *Histochem. Cytochem.* 1994;**42**:505–511.

8   Cama C, Olsson CA, Raffo AJ, *et al.* Molecular staging of prostate cancer II. A comparison of the application of an enhanced reverse transcriptase polymerase chain reaction assay for prostate specific antigen versus prostate specific membrane antigen. J Urol. 1995;**153**:1373–1378.

9   Zincke H, Oesterling JE, Blute ML, *et al.* Long term (15 years) results after radical prostatectomy for clinically localized (Stage T2c or lower) prostate cancer. J. Urol. 1994;**152**: 1850–1857.

10 Leihel SA, Zelefsky MJ, Kutcher GJ, *et al.* Three dimensional conformal radiation therapy in localized carcinoma of the prostate: interim report of phase 1 dose – escalation study. J. Urol. 1994;**152**:1792–1978.

11 Russell KJ, Caplan RJ, Laramore GE, *et al.* Photon versus fast neutron external beam radiotherapy in the treatment of locally advanced prostate cancer: results of randomized prospective trials. Int. J. *Radiation Oncology Biol. Phys.* 1993;**28**:47–54.

12 Kadmon D. Chemoprevention in prostate cancer: The role of difluoromethylornithine (DFMO). J *Cell Biochem* 1992; **16H(suppl)**:122–127.

13 Sporn MB. Chemoprevention of Cancer. *Lancet* 1993;**342**: 1211–1213.

14 Slawin K, *et al.* Dietary fenretinide, a synthetic retinoid, decreases the tumour incidence and the tumour mass of ras + myc-induced carcinomas in the mouse prostate reconstitution model system. *Cancer Res* 1993;**53**:4461–4465.

15 Hayes RB, *et al.* Serum retinol and prostate cancer. *Cancer* 1988;**62**:2021–2026.

16 Reichman ME, *et al.* Serum vitamin A and subsequent development of prostate cancer in the first National Health and Nutrition Examination Survey Epidemiologic Follow-up Study. *Cancer Res* 1990;**50**:2311–2315.

17 Rotmensz N, *et al.* Long-term tolerability of fenretinoid (4-HPR) in breast cancer patients. *Eur J Cancer* 1991;**27**: 1127–1131.

18 Hanchette CL, Schwartz GG. Geographic patterns of prostate cancer mortality: Evidence for a protective effect of ultraviolet radiation. *Cancer* 1992;**70(12)**:2861–2869.

19 Morgan RA, Anderson WF. Human gene therapy. *Ann Rev Biochem* 1993;**62**:191–217.

20 Mulligan RC. The basic science of gene therapy. *Science* 1993;**260(5110)**:926–932.

21 Hill ADK, *et al.* Cytokines in tumour therapy. *Br J Surg* 1992;**79(10)**:990–997.

22 Sanda MG, Simons JW. Gene therapy for urologic cancer. *Urology* 1994;**44**:617–624.

23 Sanda MG, Ayyagari SR, Jattee EM, *et al.* Demonstration of a rational strategy for human prostate cancer gene therapy. J. Urol. 1994;**151**: 622–628.

24 Taneja SS, Belldegrun A, de Kernion JB, *et al.* Adenoviral vector mediated high efficiency gene transfer in prostate cancer cell lines [abstract]. J *Urology* 1994;**151(5)**:253A.

25 Vieweg J, Heston WDW, Fair WR, *et al.* Use of cytokine gene-modified prostatic tumor cells for the treatment of advanced prostate cancer. J *Urology* 1994;**151(5)**:492A.

26 Isaacs WB, Carter BS, Ewing CM. Wild-type p53 suppresses growth of human prostate cancer cells containing mutant p53 allele. *Canc Res* 1992;**51(17)**:4716–4720.

27 Steiner MS, Anthony CT, Case T, *et al.* Retinoblastoma (RB) gene replacement in advanced human prostate cancer increases transforming growth factor beta-1 sensitivity and slows tumor growth. J Urol 1995;**153**:306A.

28 Yuan S, Trachtenberg J, Mills GB, *et al.* Androgen-induced inhibition of cell proliferation in an androgen-insensitive prostate cancer cell line (PC3) transfected with a human androgen receptor complementary DNA. *Canc Res* 1993;**53**:1304–1311.

29 Eastham JA, Chen SH, Sehgal I,*et al.* Prostate cancer gene therapy: HSV-tk gene transduction followed by ganeiclovin in the mouse prostate reconstitution model. J Urol 1995;**153**:307A.

30 Peng S, Sokoloff M, Teneja S. Prostate tissue-specific gene therapy utilizing a unique prostate specific antigen cytomegalovirus (PSA–CMV) promotor. J Urol 1995;**151**:307A.

31 Sokoloff M, Belldegrun A. Gene therapy for prostate cancer *Prospectives* 1995;**5**:1–8.

APPENDIX

STAGING OF PROSTATE DISEASE

Staging of Prostate Cancer		
Whitmore–Jewett	TNM 1992	Description
Incidental finding; no tumour palpable		
A1	T1a	Tumour found by chance in <5% of excised tissue
A2	T1b	Tumour found by chance in >5% of excised tissue
	T1c	Tumour confirmed by needle biopsy (raised PSA)
	Tx	Local tumour cannot be evaluated
	To	No local tumour detectable
Intracapsular palpable tumour		
B1	T2a	Tumour limited to half of one lobe or less
B2	T2b	Tumour has spread to half of one lobe but not to both
B3	T2c	Tumour has spread into both lobes
Extracapsular tumour		
C1	T3a	Unilateral extracapsular spread
C2	T3b	Bilateral extracapsular spread
	T3c	Tumour has spread to one or both seminal vesicles
	T4	Tumour is attached or has invaded adjacent structures other then the seminal vesicles
Disseminated tumour		
D1	Nx	Loco-regional lymph nodes cannot be evaluated
	N0	No lymph node involvement
	N1	Lymph nodes ≤2cm in diameter
	N2	One node only >2cm or ≤5cm; multiple ≤5cm
D2	Mx	Distant metastases can not be evaluated
	M0	No distant metastases
	M1	Distant metastases present a=lymph nodes other than regional nodes b=skeletal c=other sites
D3 resistant to hormonal therapy		

INDEX